RIVER OF STONE
RIVER OF SAND

A Story of Medicine and Adventure

RIVER OF STONE
RIVER OF SAND

A Story of Medicine and Adventure

Stephen C. Joseph, MD

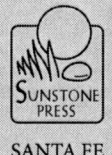

SANTA FE

All Illustrations are from the author's collection.

© 2011 by Stephen C. Joseph, MD.
All Rights Reserved.

No part of this book may be reproduced in any form or by any electronic or mechanical means including information storage and retrieval systems without permission in writing from the publisher, except by a reviewer who may quote brief passages in a review.

Sunstone books may be purchased for educational, business, or sales promotional use. For information please write: Special Markets Department, Sunstone Press, P.O. Box 2321, Santa Fe, New Mexico 87504-2321.

Book and Cover design > Vicki Ahl
Body typeface > Minion Pro
Printed on acid free paper

Library of Congress Cataloging-in-Publication Data

Joseph, Stephen C.
 River of stone, river of sand : a story of medicine and adventure / by Stephen C. Joseph.
   p. cm.
 ISBN 978-0-86534-845-5 (softcover : alk. paper)
 1. Joseph, Stephen C. 2. Physicians--Nepal--Biography. 3. Peace Corps (U.S.)--Nepal--Biography. 4. Medical assistance, American--Nepal. I. Title.
 R154.J667 2011
 610.92--dc23
 [B]
                              2011036083

WWW.SUNSTONEPRESS.COM
SUNSTONE PRESS / POST OFFICE BOX 2321 / SANTA FE, NM 87504-2321 /USA
(505) 988-4418 / ORDERS ONLY (800) 243-5644 / FAX (505) 988-1025

For Phil Lee: Teacher, Mentor, Friend

"You do not know how long you are in a river when the current moves swiftly. It seems a long time and it may be very short."

—Ernest Hemingway, *A Farewell to Arms*

PART ONE

RIVER OF STONE
NEPAL, 1964–1966

"Life is Short,
The Art Long,
Opportunity Fleeting,
Experience Treacherous,
Judgement Difficult."
—Hippocrates

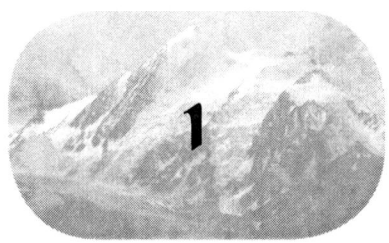

In the pre-dawn darkness, the Pan Am 'round the world Jumbo Jet lowered its flaps and backroared its way down onto the tarmac of New Delhi's International Airport. Cabin lights came on, sleep-fuggy passengers reached for coats and gear, and the forward door opened outward. Inside that door was America, and I wondered if I was leaving her behind forever. As I knelt on the economy-class seat, and stretched awkwardly up to reach the overhead bin, I tore the seat seam of my seersucker pants from stem to stern. Half-asleep, I wondered how it was going to look when, upon being initially greeted at my final destination, the mountain kingdom of Nepal, I shook hands with my right and clutched my pants together with my left. We passed quickly through the formalities of the darkened and near-deserted airport, and negotiated a taxi for the half-hour drive to Palum, the subsidiary airport from which flights departed to Kathmandu.

The air was cool but wet. A light breeze preceded dawn, with only a hint of the searing heat and choking dust of the coming August day. The bumpy tarred road had few cars or trucks at that hour, but bullock carts half-on and half-off the road slowed our progress. In the half-gray light, wraith-like figures were everywhere clad, as near as could be made out, in white robes and loincloths, squatting by the roadside or in the bushes, scurrying in and out of the gloom. Hundreds of tiny cookfires glowed like oversized candles among the trees and shadowed huts as we passed. Our headlights opened a tunnel through a phosphorescent ocean within which we seemed to glide with a constant, slow, smooth movement.

We had come from New York's Idlewild Airport through Frankfurt, Rome, and Istanbul. Now we were as if upon a different planet, headed for the still-more strange and distant asteroid of Kathmandu.

At Palum, we shuffled through one line, and then another, and then out onto the runway to board a Royal Nepal Airlines Dakota DC3. Twin-propeller workhorse of the world's backwaters, queen of a million dirt strips in a hundred thousand half-forgotten places scattered across the globe, cargo-hauler and rough-trade passenger carrier, the DC3s seemed to keep flying forever: military, civilian, smuggler, whatever was needed. There probably are still a few out there, flying on fourth-generation replacement parts. It was not the Jumbo Jet, but the Dakota, that built the Global Village.

Dawn slid under us as we winged eastward, across the sere brown summer plains of northern India. Smoke from thousands of hearths rose straight up, lazily, to meet the climbing sun, itself casting diamonds across the distant Himalayan snows. We flew on across the narrow jungle strip that forms the southern border of Nepal, and then suddenly we were flying through, and not above, gaps between green terraced ridges, their crests hanging above the level of our wings. And then, breaking through a gossamer mist, before and below us lay the Kathmandu Valley, and the immense snow peaks beyond.

It was, from the air, a child's picture book scene: the flat green, rice-paddied valley bowl, tipping up to terraced hills on all sides, with the snow mountains looming to the north. Earth-brown and cement-grey buildings clustered here and there. The valley itself lay bisected by the muddy Bagmati River. The city's structures were densely and haphazardly packed, but few buildings rose above two or three stories. As we circled closer in, one could see, fed by the maze of narrow streets, innumerable town squares, each with its multiple roof-level pagoda temple structure. Dotted here and there on the city outskirts were the dome-and-steeple *stupa* shrines. Upon the steeple base of each was painted a pair of eyes, Buddha's eyes, gazing in serene patronage over the green valley.

As the DC3 banked and swung into its approach turn, my mind's eye could see an illustration from a worn favorite book of childhood poetry, the young boy swinging up, back and forth, higher and higher, above a secret garden.

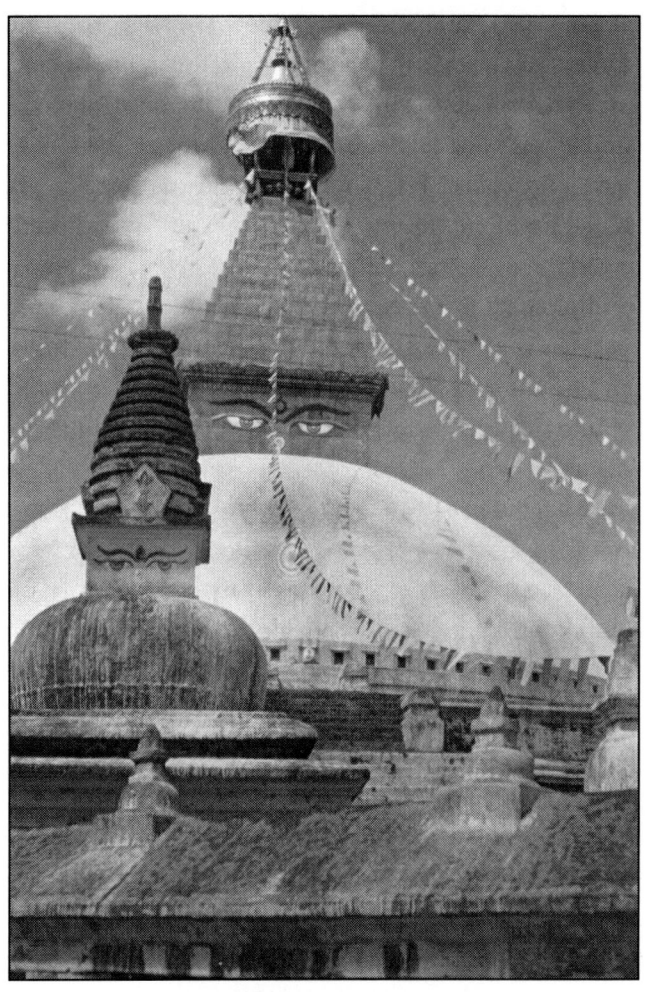

Buddhist stupas of Kathmandu valley

We bumped down onto a tar-seamed strip with a blockhouse control tower and squat terminal on one side of the runway. Thin figures pushed a baggage cart and a plain-rail staircase toward the aircraft. A small knot of individuals was standing on the tarmac. I descended the stairs, keeping my upper thighs as close together as possible under the circumstances, my small steps masking my great embarrassment.

"Hi, I'm Harry Barkely, Deputy Chief of Mission, the Ambassador's dogsbody I guess you could say. Welcome to Kathmandu, Doctor Joseph."

Harry was tall and thin, with a high forehead topped by straw-colored hair. He was New England WASP to the core. He looked straight at me and gave a firm hand. Harry was career Foreign Service, and seemed clearly destined for higher things, which he eventually achieved. As I was to learn, he did the work, ran the Embassy day to day, and was somewhat unusual for diplomats of the time in that he did not look down on the Peace Corps types as rank and bumptious amateurs. He and his wife would actually befriend the odd Volunteer who wandered in from the outlying hill country into the Big City of K'du, or he would trek out and visit them on-site in distant villages. He had a good lop-sided grin, which he tried to keep buttoned-up, but usually failed to suppress, as he had probably failed to suppress it from boyhood up through his late thirty-something years. He gave the impression of trying to be stuffy in true Brahmin (Boston, not Indian) fashion, but being equally unable to quite pull it off. Harry was completely unflapped by the flapping of my pant-sails in the prop wash, pretending not to notice at all. I, on the other hand, kept circling as we made small talk, keeping face-on to him, and was certain that I must look ridiculous.

A more chiseled and compact figure stepped forward: Willi Unsoeld, the Peace Corps Director and my new boss. "Hi, Steve, welcome. Not to rush you, but you have five or six Peace Corps patients and a couple of Embassy types wanting to see you today. Seems everybody wants to check out the new doc. We'll get you settled first, though."

Willi was of middle-size, built of some light-weight but tightly-sprung unbreakable and shiny alloy, brush-cut and with piercing blue-flint eyes. I soon learned that a year or so earlier he had temporarily left his Peace Corps job to join the first American Everest Expedition. Willi and Tom Hornbein formed the first team to reach Everest's summit via the previously-unclimbed West Ridge. They got caught in a blizzard coming down and had to bivouac overnight, up much too high and much too cold. Willi lost most of his toes, took six months or so off to recover, and then came back to his former position as Peace Corps Director, Nepal.

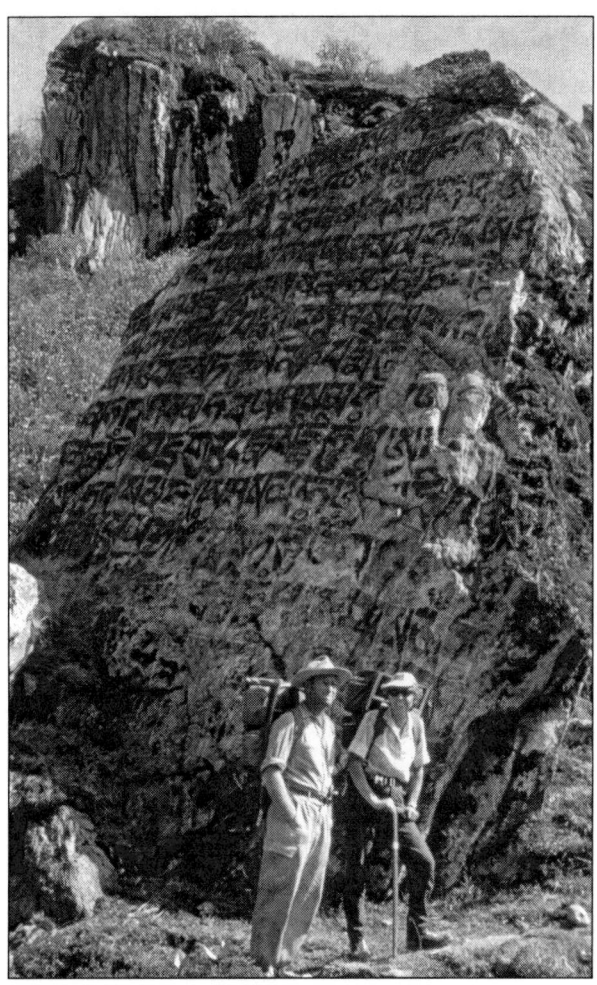

Willi and Jolene Unsoeld

There were a few other Americans from the Peace Corps staff in the greeting party, and one Nepali. He was light cherry wood skinned, with thinning white hair, fresh and trim in a suit and vest and a black short cylindrical *topi*, the national hat, worn at an angle over his smiling eyes. Dhruba Bakti, the Peace Corps office manager, fixer-upper and confessor, old enough to be the father of most of the volunteers, and father himself of the two extraordinarily beautiful daughters who were the well-guarded and unattainable delights of the dreams of all Peace Corps males. Getting anything done in Nepal was, I came to learn, a matter of *"bohli-parsi"* ("tomorrow or, perhaps, the day after tomorrow"), but if there was a way to short-circuit the system, Dhruba would know what it was, and make it work.

The small, square, two-story pink stucco house, with an upper verandah catching a view of the snow mountains, was located in the middle of a rice paddy, now rippling with tall green stalks. Several sarong-clad women curved over the plants, barefoot in the muddy water of the paddy, their bodies accenting the curve of their short sickles as they tended the ripening grain. A low-walled garden encircled the house, flowers in front and vegetables in the rear. A single-lane dirt road led from the house, winding through the paddy on a banked dike for a hundred yards or so, directly to the two-story whitewashed Peace Corps Office, which itself fronted on a tarred road heading north from the center of town. There was a telephone in the Peace Corps Office, but none in "the doctor's house." The proximity had the advantage that they always knew how to find you, and the disadvantage of being sometimes too easily reachable at any hour. This was abetted by the siting of the Peace Corps Hostel, for visiting volunteers from out-of- town or from other countries, within hailing distance of both the office and the doctor's house. It was a good setting for an old-fashioned general practice, which is what I figured I had, and what my adolescent fantasies had always wanted. A separate upstairs bedroom in the house served for taking care of those patients who were neither sick enough to be sent to the Mission Hospital across town, nor ill enough to be commercially airlifted accompanied back to the States (with me accompanying them), but who needed more medical supervision than they could get by being off on their own. A robins-egg blue, front-seat-only, soft-top jeep completed my major logistics.

And so, in Kathmandu, I began to learn how to be a doctor. I was relatively confident in my knowledge base, and I was well-supplied with books, but was I ready for the taking on of sole responsibility for my own decision process, for my own courses of action, and, ultimately, for the well-being of my patients? This was mostly new territory for me.

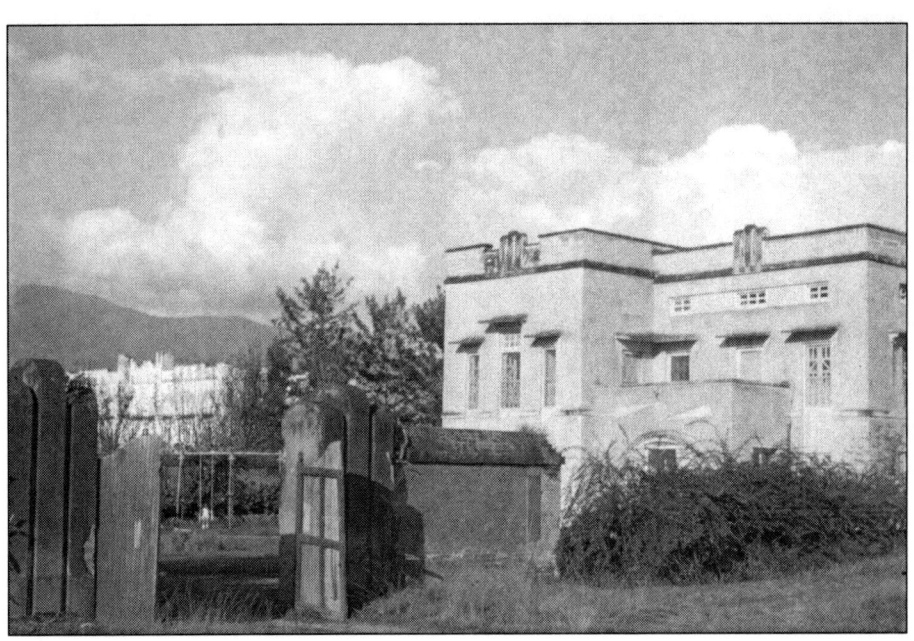

"The doctor's house"

Like countless other young physicians before and since, I began to understand that it was the *context* of my medical practice and of my relationship with my patients that was second only in importance to my skills in manipulating the physical and psychological symptoms presented for diagnosis, or the selection of appropriate medical or surgical therapy for healing. In medical training and often in medical practice in the U.S., one's patients retain a certain anonymity. Some, we get to know better over time. "Relevant medical detail," such as occupation and family history of disease, is, of course, a routine part of what we ask about their medical histories. But the context of their daily lives, and the context in which we and they live together, is not usually part of the picture we have of them, or they of us.

My situation was quite different in several important respects. My primary responsibility, the Peace Corps volunteers, were mostly young near-contemporaries of mine in age. We were part of the same organization, with a strongly shared sense of mission, and undergoing a shared experience of living in an alien, if exotic, country in which virtually everything was unfamiliar and many things virtually incomprehensible. The group was small, perhaps ninety PCVs scattered across the country, and a half-dozen staff members in Kathmandu, the capital city. There was another side, however, to this close bond of community. I was the "Company Doctor." In addition to my responsibilities for being trusted as "a good doctor" by the Peace Corps members, I also had an organizational responsibility to the program and to Willi, as its director. I had to learn to thread my way between sometimes-conflicting loyalties related to confidentiality and to best course of action.

"Doc, a bunch of us have been smoking that *ganja* marijuana over in the hostel at night. It makes me feel sick, and I'd like to stop, but I don't know how to say that to the other guys...."

"Doctor Joseph, I think I'm about three or four months pregnant. My boyfriend and I want to get married, but he's a volunteer in Senegal, and we don't finish our tours for almost another year. When I went on leave a few months ago, so did he, and we sneaked off and met for a week in Paris...."

"Steve, I just don't think I can handle it. I hate my village. It's so far away from anything I know. I'm hungry for real food all the time, can't sleep, can't concentrate, and am just sad, sad, thinking of home. The headmaster in my school where I teach tells me I'm doing a lousy job...."

I had to think long and hard about where my most relevant responsibilities lay, and how to carry them out without being disloyal or ineffective to either my patients or the program. And, in a small, close-knit community, rumors are ever present and secrets very few, whatever the geographic barriers. I knew that one major misstep, especially one that might be regarded to breach the medical confidentiality of my patients, might well render me ineffective and non-credible to the volunteers. But allowing myself to lean too far in the other direction could do significant damage to the overall accomplishments of the Peace Corps program in Nepal, and my own standing within it.

Willi, for all his charismatic leadership skills and decisive managerial efficiency, was not of much help to me in this dilemma. His views were usually more black-and-white than mine. He tended (as was probably correct from his position and perspective) to weigh the welfare of the program somewhat more than the welfare of the individual volunteer, and he was correspondingly likely to discuss the intimate issues of a volunteer with the other members of his staff. Not without significant ambivalence and discomfort, I soon learned to keep my own counsel when I judged I needed to, and to shoulder my own burdens wherever I could.

I suppose I began to develop two skills that are not taught in medical school, but become important parts of every physician's bag of tricks: the skills of evasion and the selective use of half-truths. Evasions and half-truths to ease or delay the patient's burdens of anxiety or despair. And evasions and half-truths to ease the physician's own discomfort with having to confront, and communicate, uncertainty or unwelcome news.

The setup of my medical office would not have impressed anyone at the Mayo Clinic, but to me it was ideal, and I still feel, even today, a fondness for it that surpasses that for any quarters I have worked in since. The Peace Corps building, built of unimposing gray stucco, was a two-story structure with half a third story and a water tank lumped on top, occupying a low-walled compound holding half a dozen jeeps and a small truck, fronting along the King's Road.

The ground floor was given over to storage, mailroom, Dhruba's small empire of administrative and other Nepali staff, and closets and bathrooms. The second floor contained the director's and U.S. staff offices and, along one side of its central hallway, the doctor's domain.

My consulting space was a large L-shaped room. In the main portion was my desk with its telephone, several comfortable chairs, a refrigerator for storing perishable medications and vaccines and, upon occasion, Eagle beer from India. Large windows behind my desk gave good light and sunshine to supplement the overhead lighting and floor lamps. The missing part that would otherwise square off the L, entered directly and solely from my consulting space, was a capacious stockroom for all my medical supplies. These I ordered every month from the U.S. Public Health Service Pharmaceutical Depot in Perry Point, Maryland, and a given order arrived in about four months, two months or so for supplies ordered urgently by air. I learned pretty quickly that Peace Corps/Washington did not appreciate frantic cables from feckless young doctors who had not planned ahead adequately and could not manage their pharmacy and supplies without running short of critical items.

The L-shaped portion of my office, leading off from the left end of my desk, was where the physical work got done. There was an examining table with pillow, sheets and disposable paper coverings, a movable screen behind which patients could undress, a patient measurement and weighing apparatus, a set of cabinets holding instruments, basins, and the like, and an end-wall of book shelves to hold medical and surgical texts, manuals, and whatever else I had for reading material. The only thing lacking was running water, and this was available, cold, from the staff bathroom at the end of the hall. If I needed water for what I was doing on the examining table, I would bring it in a basin, and set it on a nearby low cabinet.

As I thought about it in later years, my very first office setup in Kathmandu was not too different from what I had experienced in childhood in the late nineteen-forties, in the office of our suburban general practitioner, Dr. Irving Teitlebaum, whom I greatly admired and saw as a role model. He would talk to me about his life in medicine, and give me copies of illustrated medical throwaways sent to him by the pharmaceutical companies.

But my *real* inner sanctum and retreat was that space on the third floor, the half-floor, reached by a rickety wooden staircase from the corridor outside my office. Up there, in a converted bathroom, was my laboratory. I had a sink with running water, a tile counter with a stool, a spirit burner lamp for cooking up things, a glassware cabinet full of dishes, flasks and the like, a microscope with interchangeable lenses and its own bright light source, test tubes and racks and pipettes and glass slides and cell counting chambers, a small centrifuge, and various stains and chemicals. There was also a small autoclave for sterilizing equipment and instruments.

Up there I could immerse myself in crude but effective laboratory work. I could do red and white blood cell counts, examine urine, perform stool exams for ova and parasites (we had plenty of those), stain blood and tissue smears for bacteria and malarial and other parasites. I loved to sit up there at the end of the day after the rest of the staff had gone home and to pore over the day's specimens, teaching myself from the handbooks of clinical lab techniques and parasitology.

There were two other venues in which I could see patients. The American Embassy had a small health room, and I did most of my medical business with the diplomatic staff there, unless I needed more diagnostic or minor surgical equipment. Out beyond the edge of town, at the U.S. Agency for International Development (USAID, the foreign assistance program) compound at *Rabi Bhawan*, there was a more extensive health clinic.

During most of my time in Nepal the Embassy and USAID locales were staffed by a State Department nurse. Florence Maloney was a venerable and highly congenial old battle-axe, who had been around U.S. official expatriates for a long time in a lot of places, and who knew pretty much what there was to know about those communities. She was extremely capable, and possessed of that enthusiastic skepticism that is so valuable in general practice. We got along quite well, and I could always count on Florence if I needed an extra pair of hands, a female "observer" if I was doing a pelvic exam, or for a good chat and gossip over a hot cup of coffee. She ran the day to day business of routine care for the embassy and USAID personnel, gave the shots, kept the records, capably treated many of the medical problems, etc. When patients would bypass her and come directly to me, I would always keep her informed of what was going on with "her" patients, and this was perhaps the secret of our successful partnership. I learned much from Florence, certainly much more than she learned from me.

For a hospital base, I had the *Shanta Bhawan* United Mission Hospital. The clinical staff there was mainly American and British. Best of all, the surgeon was a young, well-trained, and highly effective American, and I never had to worry if I needed significant surgical consult help. There were x-ray and extensive clinical laboratory facilities at the hospital, and blood banking capability.

The hospital was a half-hour drive across Kathmandu from my office, and one had to cross a bridge across the Bagmati River en route. The *ghats,* or cremation platforms, lay by the river, alongside the bridge, the idea being that the ashes of the departed would wash down eventually into the holy River Ganges. Most mornings as I would cross the Bagmati on my way to see my patients, make rounds, or occasionally assist with surgery at *Shanta Bhawan*, I would make a mental note of the number and sizes of the wrapped bundles lying on the *ghats* as a sort of rough tally of how things were going in town.

Sad to say, the Nepalese government health system was in shambles. Most of the health posts and clinics in the areas outside Kathmandu were abandoned, and the major government hospital, Bir Hospital, in Kathmandu was a charnel house lacking effective care, equipment, and supplies, and was unbelievably filthy. I seldom went there, and never hospitalized patients there. Had I been a more experienced or self-assured physician, I probably would have volunteered some time at Bir and seen what I could do to help the situation, but the truth is I was not, and did not. Instead, beginning about six months after I arrived in Kathmandu, I worked with a Nepalese physician colleague at starting a maternal and child health clinic in town, an effort that moved forward in fits and starts.

I was told that off beyond the west side of Kathmandu was a small leper colony. One morning I drove my Jeep out to find it.

The rutted dirt road became a seldom-used track, and then petered out altogether. A few hundred yards beyond, against a low ridge, lay a walled compound resembling a small medieval village. Its large and sturdy gate was shut. The morning was cool and misty, and I could dimly make out robed and often-hooded figures moving both inside and outside the walls.

As I thought about walking up to that gate, I heard a tinkling bell and shuffling footsteps come from behind me. I half turned, and watched the woman approach, and then pass me on the path. She wore a thick long woolen robe in the Tibetan manner, and around her waist was the bell, hung on a woven cord, to warn others of her presence. In her arms she cradled a bundle of firewood sticks, and the left hand that held them had no fingers. I caught a half-glimpse of her face, shrouded closely by a thick woolen hood, and without taking in the specifics, I knew that the planes and angles and shadows were all wrong.

The woman passed by me without a sideward glance or a sound. Trailing along behind her was a young boy, perhaps four or five years old.

On cursory glance he appeared to be perfectly normal. I knew that I should go on and walk through that gate, to see what they needed, and what I might do. But what could I myself do? I could not obtain a long-term supply of sulfone drugs; I would not be able to *get* them to reconstructive surgery. I couldn't be there for them when they needed me.

And what about my own fear of contagion, as unlikely as that was in the short term? What about my own fears, real and otherwise?

I stood and looked at the closed gate for what seemed a long time. Then I turned back to my Jeep, and drove away.

Coward! Imposter! Are you afraid for yourself? Or are you afraid that your competence and caring would prove not adequate? Or both?

The Peace Corps volunteers who lived and worked in Kathmandu, or in the surrounding valley, or who passed through town, or came in from their stations to consult me, I saw in my office. If they needed keeping a medical eye on, they stayed in the Peace Corps hostel next door. If they needed closer medical supervision and care, I kept them in my house, in the spare bedroom. If they needed hospitalization or urgent care, there was the *Shanta Bhawan* Mission Hospital. And if they needed more sophisticated diagnostic care, or psychiatric evaluation, I put them on a plane, usually accompanying them, and flew back to the States.

There was a good deal of psychological counseling and general psychiatry involved. It was not at all uncommon for PCVs to suffer from acute depressive episodes, particularly if their work was not going well or if their isolated village-living settings were not congenial. The physician's dilemma was to try and figure out which depressions were situational and would clear rapidly, and which might be deeper and more ominous. I made hardly any use of the few anti-depressive medications that we had at the time, especially for PCVs who were in far-removed and isolated situations. Actually, those volunteers who were far away in the dramatically beautiful hill villages did, in general, much better than those who were in the urban environment of Kathmandu, or in the steamy jungles of the southern Terai flatlands. During my two years I sent or accompanied home three or four PCVs whose depressions really worried me. An observation shared by Peace Corps doctors around the world was that the level of the depression usually diminished in direct proportion to the nearer the airplane got to the U.S. I reasoned that if a PCV really didn't want to be in Nepal and under the privations and stresses of that life, it was better for them not to be there.

Nepal had the disease patterns of a very poor, highly unsanitary Third-World country, with the illnesses of both tropical and temperate climates. The volunteers, all healthy young adults to start with, and routinely immunized against everything we could think of, exhibited the patterns that one would expect: upper and lower respiratory infections, acute and chronic diarrhea and dysentery, bumps and bruises, and local minor infections of skin and eyes. There was a little bit of malaria. But there were also extremely high rates of intestinal parasites. In one group I studied, ninety percent had at least one parasite, and seventy percent had two or more. I treated many local abscesses because of lack of available hygiene, and a high rate of chronic knee problems from trekking with heavy loads. I encountered only one complicated pregnancy in a female volunteer (she was sent home), and, mercifully, no cases of active tuberculosis. Rabies was a constant worry, because of the high prevalence of rabies among the unimmunized village *pi dogs* in Nepal, and I gave a number of PCVs the dreaded series of 21 rabies shots (none in the abdomen; that was an old wives' tale by the 1960s).

Virtually every Westerner residing in Nepal who was not protected with injections of gamma globulin every six months came down with infectious hepatitis. Peace Corps policy in those days (before the shortage of gamma globulin needed for the war in South East Asia led to new studies that showed that a dose one tenth the amount that we used was equally effective) was to give such a shot, at a dose of 1 cubic centimeter per 20 pounds body weight, repeated six-monthly. That comes to 10 ccs for a large young male. If you have ever had the experience of the injection of half that amount of cold viscous material into each buttock, combined with repeated routine immunizations against plague, typhoid and paratyphoid, cholera, and whatever else Peace Corps/Washington could think of, you will understand why I was best-known, but not best-loved, for my use of the needle. The consequences of missing out on immunizations, especially the gamma globulin protection against hepatitis, could be very significant.

Only a few days after my arrival in Kathmandu I answered a knock on my front door which interrupted a quiet Sunday afternoon.

"Hi, are you the new Peace Corps doc? I just got into town, and was expecting to see Doctor Rhine."

My visitor was a tall, thin scarecrow, who said his name was Peter, and that he had flown and hitched his way up from Nepalganj, down in the Terai some two hundred miles or so away.

As my eyes adjusted to the bright sunlight, I was struck by the stained deep yellow color of his skin, and the eyeballs which fairly glowed with a similar hue.

"My gosh, Peter-whatever-your-name is, let me have a feel of your liver before I even invite you in. You look like the Peace Corps poster boy for hepatitis. How long have you been sick, and when was your last gamma globulin shot? Anyway, my name is Steve Joseph, and won't you come in."

I regained my professional composure, such as it was, got him inside, took the typical history to go along with his jaundice and his enlarged tender liver, and heard his sheepish explanation that he had been "too busy" to make sure he had gotten his gamma globulin for a year or more.

There really wasn't much medically to do. What he needed was rest, an adequate and appropriate diet, and careful watching. So Peter became the first patient I "hospitalized" in our spare bedroom, and our first houseguest, all at the same time. He did fine, went back to serve out his tour in Nepalganj, and eventually became the American Ambassador to a country in Asia.

Much of my Peace Corps practice, unlike that of a doctor in the States, was heavily dependent upon, and complicated by, issues of logistics and communications. For the volunteers in the Kathmandu Valley, this was not unusually difficult, except for the scarcity of telephones and automobile transport.

For those volunteers further afield, and that was most of them, the situation was quite different. On average, these PCVs were a week or more distant by foot from Kathmandu, and most of them were a two days or so trek from a grass airstrip with service to the capitol. There were no telephones, and in very few cases were there nearby missionary health services. In many, if not most, instances, communication between the volunteers and me regarding acute or emergent problems depended upon either the government wireless telegram system, or upon the volunteer just showing up at my office or home door, after long and arduous travel.

The wireless was itself plagued by delay, ambiguity, and uncertainty. The volunteer would have to reach the nearest station, which might be a day's walk from his or her home village. Though the PCVs all spoke good Nepali, a medical message would have to be transliterated from English (which virtually none of the wireless operators spoke) into written Nepali (which uses a Sanskrit-based alphabet), sent to Kathmandu Central, delivered to the Peace Corps office, and then transliterated back into English. One can imagine the potentials for error and uncertainty in such a system. Most importantly, the average time for a wireless message sent to me was often as much as four to five days from sending to receiving. If I wanted to send a message back asking for further information or giving medical instruction, it would take a similar amount of time to reach the volunteer. This, of course, was untenable if the situation seemed to be one of acute or emergency need. Thus much of my practice involved trying to decide or intuit whether to make emergency trips by commercial aircraft, or by fixed wing or helicopter assets of the Embassy, out to visit the PCV on-site.

Volunteers were furnished with an extensive medical kit, much more elaborate than the usual "patch and smear" variety one thinks of. They also had stool sample kits which could be sent in to me by whatever means were available. I also found a routine letter system very useful: pre-stamped and pre-addressed mailgrams were sent in monthly to Kathmandu by each volunteer, directly and confidentially to me, in which any medical problems, any needs for medical re-supply, or anything else the volunteer might want me to know or to communicate to the other staff members, could be related. This would often give me a head's up on developing medical or social problems, and provide a way for my patients and me to have a continuing relationship, even at long distance and long-delayed intervals. Some of those mailgrams would arrive weeks or months after sending. The mailgram system also helped me to plan my travel schedule, and to carry out to distant volunteers those small personal items, as well as mail from home, that are so all-important to the morale of those in isolated and difficult environments.

It was a toss-up whether the largest elements of my Peace Corps practice were psychological or gastrointestinal, and indeed the two areas were often linked, either in psychosomatic or reactive fashion. Diarrhea and dysentery, dysentery and diarrhea: acute episodes, chronic distress, weight loss, nausea and vomiting. There were viral and bacterial causes, and a wealth, if that word is appropriate here, of parasitic ones: amoebas, worms of a wide variety, and those stubborn cases that resisted all my clinical and laboratory efforts at diagnosis. I learned that a careful and exhaustive history was usually of more help than physical examination. When repeated laboratory examinations yielded no answers, I learned that blind therapeutic trials sometimes led to astounding success, and upon occasion to totally unwarranted praise.

The diet, for rural volunteers especially, was a monotonous and bulky rice and lentil *dal bhat*, with only very occasional meat or chicken or fresh vegetables. A curious but very dependable finding was that male PCVs lost weight, sometimes to considerable extent, and that female PCVs gained excessive and unhealthy weight. I never achieved a satisfactory explanation of this phenomenon. Chronic diarrhea would thin any of them down, and sometimes the most important physical and psychological benefits of "hospitalizing" volunteers in my house for a week or so came from just feeding them up on the more appetizing and varied diet we could find and afford in Kathmandu. The amount of food that some of them could pack away in those circumstances was a constant source of amazement to my cook.

I treated a lot of insignificant respiratory infections, the occasional pneumonia, skin rashes and superficial fungal junk, lots of bumps and bruises and sprains, and the occasional significant laceration or minor fracture. I lanced more boils and abscesses than I can remember, pierced a fair number of female ear lobes (after all, better me with sterile equipment and technique than the guy on the street corner with unwashed hands and dirty needles), and enjoyed the this and that of which much small town practice is composed. I treated a number of cases of gonorrhea, but never had a PCV with syphilis.

I had been in Kathmandu for about two weeks, getting myself organized, beginning to work out some comfortable routines, getting to know the Peace Corps staff and local volunteers, when Willi appeared in my office door one morning.

"Steve, it's probably time to get you on the road, get some blisters on your heels, and have you begin to learn what this country is really about. Don Mussler, who works on community development in Kuncha, is heading back out there from K'du in a day or so, and he would be a good guide on your first trail trip, which ought to be an easy one. I'll send him by to see you later today, and you two can talk it over. Don't forget to take plenty of moleskin for your tender tootsies."

Don was a burly, bluff, Alaskan, with lots of outdoor experience, and a full year as a volunteer in the Central Hills under his belt.

We chatted a bit, and Don said, "How about if we travel together to my place in Kuncha. This will get you started, and then you could go on alone for a last stage of two or three days to Pokhara, the largest town west of Kathmandu in the Central Hills."

"That sounds like a good idea," I replied. "I know that there are several households of PCVs in Pokhara, and that itinerary would give me a good start on familiarizing myself with a key route and on learning to travel in Nepal."

In those days there were three ways you could get directly to Pokhara from Kathmandu. You could walk for five days. You could fly Royal Nepal directly or with an intermediate stop at the grass airstrip near Ghorka, at a place called Palungtar, mid-way in between. Or, as Don and I were planning, you could fly to Gorkha and then walk the final two days into Pokhara. There were no motorable roads west out of the Kathmandu Valley, and none coming east out of Pokhara. The trip was a classic Nepal journey, except for the lack of any particularly difficult river crossings or big ridge climbs along the way. It was a good start for a tenderfoot, as Willi no doubt had in mind.

Don helped me plan to fill my pack with what I would need to sleep, eat, and keep going on the trail. "This is still monsoon season, so we didn't need to worry about cold, but we do need to be able to keep ourselves, and especially our feet, dry. So, most of your spare clothing should be socks. In Nepal, you can always find a place to sleep: a friendly farmer will offer you a porch or a corner of a room in a village you are passing through. There is never a need for a tent. Forget about an air mattress, so that cuts the sleeping issue down to a light bag, and, if you are really fussy, a light but waterproof groundsheet. Eating is likewise a matter of asking for a place at a villager's simple meal. And, by the way, it's considered very bad manners to offer to pay for the meal until you leave the next morning. You can almost always buy tea, biscuits, or rice at a local tea house along the trail. That cuts down the food you have to carry to snacks and a few dry rations. You'll never need to take a stove or eating utensils. Everybody eats with their fingers. Well, if you're fussy enough to take a groundsheet, you might even roll a spoon up in it. All in all, what you need is a sleeping bag, your spare clothes and washing-up gear (including a flattened half-roll of toilet paper), a poncho in monsoon season, flashlight, knife, fire-making materials, a few personal odds and ends, whatever map you have, and that's pretty much it. And, oh yes, you need a canteen and iodine tablets to disinfect the universally contaminated water. The trail system in Nepal is what you follow, asking the way from one village to the next along your route. So, most of the time, once you get the hang of it, you don't even need a map, not really."

"What about a compass, Don?"

"Very few of us carry. Since the trails had been developed and used for hundreds of years, they always follow the best walking route from one place to another, and there's no point in ever bushwhacking across country. Some volunteers walk, Nepali-style, with a rolled umbrella for a walking stick. One more tip, throw a hundred feet of parachute cord in your pack; it has a thousand uses. Not too complicated, but don't forget the extra socks."

I learned that a well-organized volunteer could keep the pack down to under twenty pounds. I, however, had a different problem. I had to figure out how to carry, in addition to my regular load, an adequate medical kit, and it took me many months to work out how to fit the maximum range and quantity of items I wanted to have with me into the minimum weight and volume. I never did get my load down below fifty, sometimes even sixty, pounds, and though this got me into great trail shape, it was a constant struggle to find another ounce or two that I thought I could give up. I learned from Willi, whose obsessive-compulsive-ness put mine to shame, that no tiny amount was too small to strip away. For me, this included tossing out the printed package inserts and cardboard coverings on medicines, cutting off the long loose ends of syringe envelopes, and the like. Willi had two rules I adopted: "Never take a step down when you are climbing up, and never carry an ounce that you can do without." After all, ounces turn into pounds, and every pound you don't have to carry, up hill and down, for days or weeks, takes a bit of load off your back and your feet.

The standard issue Peace Corps pack was nothing special, but Willi had gotten his hands on a small number of the (then) new Kelty frame packs, which he allowed people to use only with his special permission. Dhruba, bless his soul, finagled one for my personal possession. I loved that huge old green square monster; it stood up well above my head when I threw it on and buckled the high waist strap, but it was capacious as an old-time steamer trunk, and its design and weight-distributing characteristics were then the latest thing in outdoor gear. As soon as I got back to the States at the end of my tour I bought myself another one, and I still have it, forty years later, though it looks like a Model-T in comparison to contemporary pack designs. It was tall and rectangular, with an oversized pull-down top cover to the main compartment, allowing me to stuff stuff, so to speak, beyond the capacity of the compartment itself. There were five big zippered additional pockets, one on the front and two on each side, and an empty space along the bottom of the external frame, below the main compartment, where I could strap on a sleeping bag or other bulky gear. The Kelty's major problem was size and balance when going along a narrow trail, say in thick forest or along a cliff face with an overhang on the uphill side. You could get swept off your feet if you weren't careful. The only thing that the Kelty lacked, as did all trail transport in Nepal, was wheels.

When I had followed Don's advice about Spartan packing for the Nepal Hills, and then, on this first trip, added all the medical supplies and equipment I could cram in, he didn't offer any comment. But he looked me up and down, and then spent a long minute staring at my feet, and the message was obvious: "You and your feet are in for a surprise, Greenhorn."

Don and I took the afternoon DC3 from Kathmandu airport. This plane did not have the usual rows of passenger seats, just a ledge of tube and webbing seating running lengthwise along each side of the fuselage. Freight was tied down under cargo nets along the center of the aircraft. Two Nepali women and their babies were the only other passengers on our flight, and they clutched each other, cowering on the center floor, holding on to the tie-downs, and shaking as the DC3 revved its engines and taxied down the runway.

We flew west, low along the green valleys, at right angles to the rising ridges and parallel to the snow mountains beyond to the north, at this season encircled by heavy afternoon clouds. In less than thirty minutes we swung into the grass airstrip at Palungtar, on a wide flat area below the climb to the village of Ghorka on the ridge above. A pole and leaf lean-to at one side of the field was the only administrative or passenger waiting area at Palungtar. Ticket processing and loading was done by the pilot and co-pilot on the flights landing and taking off. There were about four takeoffs or landings a day, half going on to Pokhara, and half returning to Kathmandu. In the months to follow, I was to fly in and out of Palungtar many times. If a plane didn't arrive, heading in the direction I wanted to go, I just waited, sometimes for several days, until one did, or, if the weather was obviously down for a day or so, climbed two hours up the ridge to wait in Ghorka.

There was a very small mission hospital, more like an expanded clinic, in Ghorka, and Don introduced me to the woman who was the entire medical staff. She had one patient in the house at that time, a man dying of rabies. The Ghorka area was currently experiencing an outbreak of dog rabies, something not unusual in Nepal, and there were several humans who had been bitten and infected. There had never been, at that date, a known human survivor of rabies once symptoms developed, and it was, to doctors and communities alike, a most terrifying disease.

The patient that I saw, actually the only human case of rabies I have ever seen, was heavily sedated, but still having periodic convulsions. The clinic at Ghorka had no supply of rabies vaccine, and thus anyone bitten by a suspect dog, or an animal who then escaped capture, just had to wait it out and take their chances. Either they would remain healthy, or develop symptoms and die a horrible death. After watching the death struggles of the patient at Ghorka, I hope never to see another case.

That early experience made me an arch-conservative in insisting that volunteers, or anyone else, who were bitten or scratched by an animal that could not be positively established as having been vaccinated against rabies (and that was pretty much every animal in Nepal, except for a few pets of Western expatriates in Kathmandu), receive a full course of rabies vaccine. As you might imagine, I used a large amount of vaccine. I would sometimes make an exception of shortening the course of injections if the animal could be kept and observed for a week or more without showing symptoms of illness.

It never ceased to amaze me how people would come up with arguments to try and avoid twenty-one injections, where there was otherwise even the small possibility of an outcome of certain, and particularly disagreeable, death. It was an early important lesson to me concerning the strong predilection of humans to go to extraordinary lengths to convince themselves of what they wish to believe with regard to medical matters.

We shared the doctor's simple meal of *dal bhat*, passed a comfortable night sleeping on her front porch, and made the two- or three-hour trek over to Kuncha early the next morning. I spent the rest of the day with Don and his village-mate, Bruce, treated a few minor illnesses among the Kuncha villagers, and the next morning I took off for Pokhara, alone for the first time in the Nepal Hills.

It was not a difficult walk. I discovered that my Nepali, though halting, was adequate to ask the way if I was uncertain, got wet a couple of times in monsoon showers, and was able to get myself fed and housed trailside. The trails were wet and, nearer to Pokhara, sometimes water covered in this season, and I had my share of greenhorn's blisters on my heels and between my toes by the time I arrived in town.

In those days, when a Westerner arrived in a village, even a town as large as Pokhara, with a pack on his or her back, everyone knew who you were and who you were looking for. When you asked the way to the *Peace Corps manche*, children would fall in beside you, or take you by the hand, singing and laughing, and lead you to the volunteers' house.

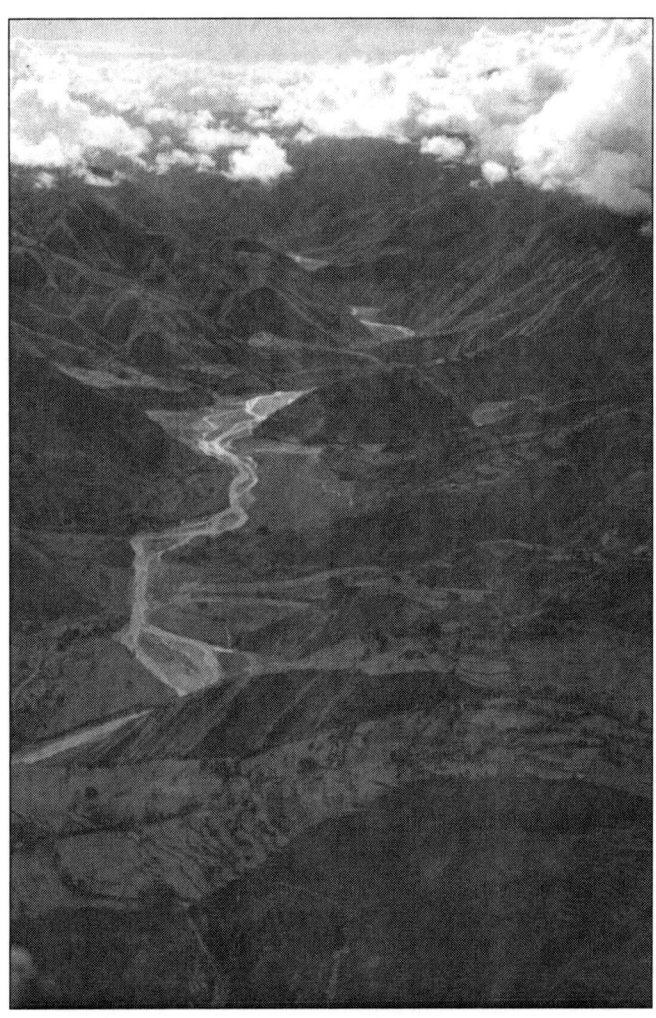

Valley trail to Pokhara

When I reached the first house, I found a group of very worried volunteers gathered and awaiting me. They had known that I was coming, from a wireless telegram that had been sent days before I left Kathmandu. But two days before I arrived in Pokhara, in other words on the morning that I had left Kuncha, an urgent message had been received, hand-delivered from the airport.

REGRET INFORM DOCTOR THAT PCV ANDREW GRAY REPORTED KILLED IN FALL FROM TRAIL THIRTY SIX HOURS PREVIOUSLY STOP ACCIDENT OCCURRED WHILE TREKKING AT NIGHT ALONG DUDH KHOSI STOP NO FURTHER CURRENT DETAILS STOP PC STAFF ENROUTE HELICOPTER EVAC BODY TO KATHMANDU FOR TRANSPORT HOME TO STATES END

I learned from the other volunteers that Andy was a popular and competent community development worker over in the eastern part of the country, far in the opposite direction from Kathmandu from where I now was. This was the first death of a PCV in Nepal, and hit everyone extremely hard.

I had a truncated visit with the Pokhara volunteers, did the minimum of necessary medical business with them, and rushed early the next morning down to the Pokhara airstrip, beyond the far southern end of town, to catch the mid-day flight back to Kathmandu, making a brief stop, ironically, at Palungtar along the way.

By the time I got back to Kathmandu, the body had been recovered, placed in a sealed metal casket, and was on a commercial flight back to the States. I was shaken by the episode, and spent many hours thinking through the implications. First, it imprinted upon me how likely it was that important medical issues could arise in which I could play no part at all, given the difficulty of communications and logistics in Nepal. I kept thinking that, although I could have done nothing to alter the outcome in this case, I *should have been there*, to deal with the issues of retrieving the body, to be, as the doctor, available to volunteers and staff, to take responsibility for dealing with the legal complexities of flying the body home, etc. However irrationally, I was unable to shake the feeling that I hadn't done my job.

But, more importantly, suppose the accident had not led to an immediate fatality? What if emergency medical care had been needed, trailside or in the nearest village? What if death or irreversible injury took place twenty-four or forty-eight hours later? How *could* I do my job, given the hours and days it would take to become aware and then respond?

Thus, what could have been an easy introduction into my work outside Kathmandu turned into the darkest days of my first year in Nepal.

I wondered if I was up to the job, or if indeed the job was possible to do.

I wondered whether I would perform appropriately when the next, and inevitable, emergency-at-a-distance arose.

I wondered whether I would over-react from this point forward, seeing emergencies where there weren't any. And how could I tell the difference, anyway?

And then I finally realized that I wasn't in Boston any more, and that I had better get on with figuring out, to the extent I could, how to do the best I could with what I had.

Many volunteers stationed in other countries in Asia or even elsewhere wandered into Kathmandu, either during a period of leave or on a world-journey at the conclusion of their service. Most of them stayed in the Peace Corps hostel, most of them got sick with diarrhea, and most of them came to see me. Occasionally, I would encounter a real diagnostic puzzle in some ex-PCV who had left another country three months earlier, and presented in Kathmandu with a chronic health problem.

The situation of recently-discharged volunteers presented me with the worst problem, and the most damage, not deliberate, of course, that I ever inflicted on a volunteer in Nepal. It happened this way:

When a volunteer's two-year assignment was up, he or she had a choice: they could return directly to the States by air, or they could request the equivalent air fare and go wherever they wished, at their own pace and itinerary. This latter was favored by most volunteers, as it gave them an opportunity to "see the world" at little expense.

There was one catch, however. At administration "termination" of a particular group, every PCV went through a full medical exam, including basic laboratory studies. If a readily and rapidly treatable condition could be satisfactorily dealt with in-country, there was no problem. They got treated, and then were administratively "terminated." But, if a more complicated issue arose, or if specialized or lengthy diagnosis or treatment was necessary, then the rules were that the PCV was to be returned directly to Washington for processing and termination.

Bill and Jane were a young married couple who had had a rough tour. They had been posted as schoolteachers in the hot and sweaty Terai, and I had seen them repeatedly for gastrointestinal problems. Their school headmaster was hostile to them, their living situation was difficult, but they had stuck it out, not without significant strain on the marriage. A major factor in their perseverance was the six-month long "dream trip" that they had been planning to undertake, back through the Middle East and then Europe, at the end of their two years of service.

After the usual discussion and physical exam, I called them back when their lab results returned from the hospital.

"Bill, Jane, you know that almost everyone of the volunteers has intestinal parasites whenever we check for them. Most of them are quite easily treated, but not all. Bill, you have some garden-variety roundworms, and we can take care of that quickly. A bit disgusting, but no problem. But Jane, your stool exam shows that you have a tapeworm. I don't see that very often in volunteers, but there it was, and we need to get rid of it."

"What's the problem? Is the treatment difficult or dangerous? How long will it take? We plan to fly out of Kathmandu next week, starting our trip."

"Well, it shouldn't be the treatment that is the problem. We have one drug, Atabrine, which you take by mouth. It can temporarily give your skin a yellow color, but other side effects are rare. The key is to keep checking your stools during and after treatment, to make sure that you pass all of the worm, including its tiny head segment. If you don't get rid of that, the nasty critter just goes ahead and grows more segments."

"How long should the process of treatment and cure take?"

"That, I'm afraid, is the problem. It should only take about a week or ten days, but the rule-book says that I'm supposed to return you direct to Washington for this, and have you get medically-terminated after successful treatment there."

"What! No, Doc, you can't do that. You know about this trip we've been planning for over a year now. We just…." Jane was stammering, and I noticed that Bill let go of her hand and just shifted his weight slightly away from her chair next to his.

We talked about it for a while. In the end I just couldn't bring myself to do what the procedures told me I should do. So I put Jane into *Shanta Bhawan*, not because of any medical risk, but because it was easier to make sure we got 100% of the messy business of examining all stools done right. We retrieved the worm's head, Jane seemed normal, and they and I were equally relieved to see them board that airplane, free as birds.

Three weeks later I received a cable from the Peace Corps doctors in Turkey:

> DO YOU HAVE KNOWLEDGE OR RECORDS RE. FORMER NEPAL PCV JANE SMITH STOP SUBJECT APPARENTLY IN PSYCHIATRIC HOSPITAL IN IZMIR RECEIVING ELECTROSHOCK TREATMENT FROM TURKISH MD STOP ALLEGEDLY DEEPLY JAUNDICED STOP PLEASE ADVISE STAT END.

Ask any GI who was in the Pacific in World War Two: Atabrine, then in use as a synthetic anti-malarial, can turn you yellow, as I had mentioned to Bill and Jane. Medical people know that there is also a rare and temporary side effect in some cases, called "Atabrine psychosis." I had dropped the ball: deliberately not followed proper Peace Corps procedures, but, more important, not warned the Smiths adequately about the very small risk of serious side effects. Worse than the self-limited side effects was that Jane was now in some hell-hole in southern Turkey getting electroshock therapy. My colleagues got her out of there (we were not supposed to have any responsibility for former Volunteers wandering the world, but of course we all did everything and anything we could for all of them, whatever the regulations). It turned out all right in the end, but I felt deeply, and still do, about my part in the episode.

I had a serious trading relationship with the Peace Corps doctor in Thailand, an extremely able, and, by all accounts, pleasant woman. It was in the nature of things that many male PCVs would go to Thailand on leave, and amongst the cultural splendors of Bangkok get their ashes hauled in ways and to extents that were difficult to come by in Nepal. Conversely, Thailand PCVs were anxious to come to the fabled and romantic Himalayas, trek and climb the mountains, and obtain temporary relief from the muggy heat of

Thailand. They all developed intestinal problems from the contaminated food and water of Nepal.

So, I got to treat all of Doctor Martha's g.i. problems, and she got to treat all of my venereal disease, and then we got to reverse the process when our respective volunteers returned to their stations. We had quite a nice relationship, though we never met in person.

A classic Peace Corps story concerns the Peace Corps hostel in Bangkok, and illustrates the complexity of communication and logistics of the period. Literally hundreds of current and recently discharged volunteers would pass through the Bangkok hostel, on their way to all parts of the globe. One day, an urgent cable from Peace Corps/Washington was sent to all posts:

> RABIES CONFIRMED IN DOG RESIDENT IN PC/THAILAND HOSTEL BETWEEN DATES JUNE 15-JULY 15 APPROXIMATE STOP PLEASE ASCERTAIN ANY YOUR PCV'S IN HOSTEL DURING THAT PERIOD AND IMMUNIZE ANY WHO MAY HAVE HAD DIRECT CONTACT WITH SUCH AN ANIMAL STOP ADVISE PC/WASH ANY SUCH ACTION END

This was clearly an impossible instruction to carry out fully, but what else was Peace Corps to do? The consequences of missing the chance to prevent a fatal case of rabies in a volunteer would have been catastrophic. Fortunately, no case ever occurred. But Peace Corps doctors all over the world scrambled through leave records for dates and destinations, contacted the relevant PCVs, etc. I had four volunteers in Nepal who were "possibles" by date and location, but none of them reported being scratched or bitten, or even remembered the dog. But still I worried.

It was, of course, impossible to track *former, recently-discharged* volunteers who had passed through Bangkok on an extended journey home.

Among the more serious things I dealt with among the volunteers were the occasional cases of amoebic dysentery, infectious hepatitis in volunteers who were not up to date on their gamma globulin, and one or two scarily severe cases of malaria. There were a couple of severe acute depressions that I thought might be psychotic and that took me some time to organize for evacuation to the States, while I kept the agitated patient sedated with Thorazine in Kathmandu.

What I feared most, but never saw in the volunteers, was active tuberculosis (rampant in Nepal), attack by a rabid dog (ditto), and, because of the experience on my initial trek into the Hills, extensive and life-threatening trauma or medical emergency at a distance that I couldn't get to in time.

And, at the bottom line, that was the biggest difference between what I was learning, and what most young doctors at my stage of development were learning. For most of them, it was a matter of "it", bad as it might be, coming to them. For me, it was a matter of me being able to get to "it." That's what kept me awake at night, and led to endless scheming and worrying regarding ways to improve and shorten communication, logistics, and transportation.

There were several other components of my practice, beyond the Peace Corps volunteers, that added immeasurably to my pleasure and education. Beyond the official American community there were expatriates of all varieties, many of them interesting people doing interesting things. I had a nice general practice among them, for even if it was clear to all concerned that I was in no way what my parents liked to call "a Very Big Doctor", I was a very scarce commodity in town, and people came to me in significant numbers. I also regularly made house calls, which is an experience that every young doctor should have. I could not and would not charge for my services, but some people insisted in paying in chickens or small gifts. The most important currency, of course, was lots of friendship and goodwill, and also informal access to returned favors and information. But, I must admit, there is something very nice about being paid in the occasional chicken, or, as I have in other circumstances, in the gift of a fresh-caught salmon. It takes medicine, at least for this incurable romantic, back to a time and place that has a different, and closer, emotional bond between physician and patient.

David Abraham was the young Rockefeller Foundation representative in Kathmandu, and, like many of my expatriate patients, a friend of mine. One morning he appeared at my office door, frightened and very anxious. In tow was his eleven-year-old daughter, Rosalie, whose eyeballs and skin were stained a deep yellow.

"Steve, I took Rosalie to a Nepali doctor in town. He says she has hepatitis. But she has gotten all her gamma globulin shots. She seems weak and tired, but otherwise well. What's going on?"

"C'mon, Sweetie," I said, winking at Rosalie. "Let me poke around your tummy gently a little bit, and look in your beautiful eyes. You know I won't hurt you."

On examining Rosalie, I found neither an enlarged nor tender liver. She was obviously jaundiced, but she looked to me to also be very anemic, and quick tests in my upstairs lab proved this to be the case.

"Dave, I don't think Rosalie has hepatitis, or one of the various things that can cause obstructive jaundice. It seems to me that the most likely thing is that she is hemolysing—breaking down her red blood cells in large amounts, possible due to some sort of toxic reaction. Has she been exposed to any chemicals or unusual substances in the past few days?"

"The beans, Daddy, the beans, just like Granma said!" Rosalie exclaimed.

"In response to my quizzical look, David replied, "That's right. My mother, who as you know lives with us, saw Rosalie and me eating some beans off the tree in our yard last weekend."

"David, go get Rosalie's grandmother and come back as quick as you can."

The old lady, whose Arabic was better than her English, explained patiently that everybody knew, where she grew up in the Jewish community in Lebanon, that *bachooli* beans could make some people turn yellow. Her own mother, who came originally from Baghdad, had taught her that.

I dug through my now-worn copy of Manson's *Tropical Diseases*. It turns out that the Jewish community in Baghdad, resident there since the Old Testament time of the Babylonian captivity, had the world's highest prevalence of a congenital enzymatic defect that caused them to undergo significant hemolysis when exposed to certain agents, including the fava beans of the so-called *bachooli* tree.

Rosalie recovered rapidly without incident, never needing transfusion. When the Abrahams went on home leave to the States, I sent my case notes with them, and the local medical school in Tennessee confirmed the diagnosis of congenital G-6-PD deficiency. The benefit of all this was that she and her family now knew that she had it, and were aware of a number of medicines and other substances, including fava beans, that she had to avoid.

Fabulous! From Ancient Babylon to Baghdad to Beirut to Kathmandu to Tennessee. Always cherchez la Grandmere if you want to make the diagnosis!

Beyond the expatriates, my more important medical practice was among the Nepalis, and it took place more often outside Kathmandu, during my travels in the Hills. Here I would hold roving clinics while visiting volunteers, taking on all comers in whatever ways I could.

I developed a friendship with a missionary doctor who had a small but well-equipped solo operation at the far eastern edge of the Kathmandu Valley, out near Banepa. The jeep road from K'du ended there, and the foot trails in the Hills began. On several occasions when Keith left his hospital for a short period to attend a conference in India, or took some much-deserved brief leave, he asked me to come out and cover for him. I was only too glad to do so, and attend to his in-patients, deliver a baby or two, and run his dispensary, minor surgery, and mobile clinics with the experienced help of his well-trained Nepali nurses. It was only about an hour's rough drive from Banepa back to the Peace Corps office, and I could manage to keep in reasonable touch with things for a few days or a week. Keith had a comfortable bungalow, and a well-stocked library. I would spend my late evenings reading through his texts, especially the well-illustrated ones on general practice, listening to his medical audiotapes. During those pleasant evenings and long nights, I feared, more than anyone could imagine, the knock on the door that would announce a true surgical emergency in the chest or belly, which I was in no way adequately prepared to deal with. I figured that his Nepali surgical assistant could get me through it if it came, but it never did. I had tremendous admiration and respect for Keith, working year after year, on his own, doing what he could , which was very substantial, with what he had, which wasn't much.

And then there were my non-human patients. People would ask me to see dogs and cats and all sorts of critters, most of them beloved pets. There was in effect no veterinary service available, and so they came to me, the next best thing.

Willi had a German Shepherd, named Katie, a *really* big and imposing watchdog. When she developed a nasty abscess in her outer ear canal, he asked me to do something about it. She was obviously in pain, and I worried that she might be extra-irritable. I approached her with some caution, holding out my hand, palm up, and saying the Nepali equivalent of "nice dog." It is true that we knew each other, but I was amazed when Katie jumped up on the pantry table, lay over on her side, and let me examine and treat her without any resistance. I sprayed some ethyl chloride on the mass to freeze it, incised it, cleaned it out, and stuck on a wick and dressing. Katie jumped down from the table, wagged her tail, and that was it.

I had car-struck dogs that needed to be put down (that, let me tell you, is painful work), goats, a monkey or two, and even the housecat of the king's brother's American mistress, who had a skin rash (the cat, not the mistress). And chickens. I did not do very well with chickens, nor with parakeets, for that matter. When a virus gets into a small flock, at least in my experience, it is Goodbye Charlie.

Ever since I had been an early adolescent quizzing Dr. Teitlebaum or thumbing through, over and over, the *Life Magazine* photo essay about the solo general practitioner in small-town Colorado, I had wanted some version of what I now found myself experiencing in Nepal. Pretty much on my own, surrounded by mountains, trying to figure out how to do what I could with what I had. It hadn't been very hard getting here, but being here, being able to do what I depended on myself to do, and what others depended on me for, was proving much harder. I wouldn't have traded it for anything.

2

The road that had brought me to Nepal, arriving in Kathmandu that morning of August 11, 1964, had begun much earlier, stretching back even beyond my youthful summers in the Shining Mountains of Wyoming, and on through my years in medical school. But it had really begun to take specific shape during the early weeks of my internship, just a year before that morning of my arrival at the Kathmandu airport.

While in medical school I had found myself drawn to pediatrics. Later in life it would seem to me that my personality, even back then, would have been better suited to the bang-bang of trauma surgery, or to one of the yet-to-be defined specialties of emergency medicine or sports medicine. While one large part of me was undoubtedly an adrenaline junkie, and still is, I found myself drawn to the puzzling-out of children, especially to the black boxes of neonates and infants. Trying to learn to see the world through another culture's eyes, the culture of childhood, learning to not only speak through the intermediaries of parents, but to attempt to communicate *directly* across an unbridgeable frontier with a sick child, held a fascination for me.

There was another, more selfish, reason as well, one that increasingly took shape as my medical education progressed.

I knew that I was not much interested in well children. I liked, if I may put it this way, really sick kids, kids on the edge, the more desperately ill the better. Give me a fifteen-month old, red-hot with sepsis or meningitis, rolling into the emergency room at three in the morning, that is what lit up my bulbs.

My favorite internship rotations were the acute care wards, the emergency room, and, especially, the surgical emergency room. On the days when Dr. Samuel Katz, the Chief of Infectious Disease, was giving teaching rounds on the wards, I would rush through my outpatient clinic appointments and steal away upstairs, standing at the back of the white-coated crowd, hanging on his every word.

I knew I was not headed for a suburban middle-class practice where I would burn out in no time at all, nor for a research career, as I knew from early days on that I didn't have the focused intellectual horsepower to compete successfully in that arena. I wanted to spend my time, at least as far ahead as I could look, which was not very far nor well-thought out, in the wild and untrammeled places of the world, close up to the natural mysteries that had opened to me in the Shining Mountains of Wyoming. So I set my sights, in some vague and unplanned way, on what was then called "tropical pediatrics." As I saw it, that was where the most dramatic and intractable medical problems were; that's where the resources were scarcest; and that's where, in some naïve way, I figured that I could be in the life-environment I wanted, doing what I could with what I had. There were little or no political, altruistic nor "missionary" aspects to the calculus; it just seemed to be what would fit me best, to the extent that I could look into the future further on than a year or so. "Plan ahead" has never been my strong suit, and still is not.

I began my internship in the summer of 1963 in an academic setting in a Boston teaching hospital. I dove into it, ferociously, devouring as much as my mind and body could encompass, neglecting family, friends, and any other interests, just wanting more and more of that indescribably-alive first experience of learning to practice medicine.

In those days we worked hard in ways that are now politically incorrect and that seem, by today's standards, inadequately supervised. It was standard practice that interns, and most residents, worked shifts of "every other night and every other weekend." This meant that, all year long, you came on duty about 7 am Monday, went home about 7pm Tuesday, and laid your body down little or not at all in between. Then you started again about 7am Wednesday, and had Thursday and Friday nights off, if you could get your work cleared up, before coming in early Saturday morning to work straight through until Monday evening. Then you would start the opposite weekly shift: Monday and Wednesday nights off, but then on duty from Thursday morning until Saturday afternoon, when you got off until Monday morning. Thus the cycle of the year was spent in a strange combination of exhilaration and chronic exhaustion.

One anecdote will suffice. I remember dropping into bed in my hospital on-call room about two in the morning. The next thing I remember, as if still in a dream, I was standing, fully-dressed, on the ward, at the nursing station, finishing writing up my notes and orders on an acutely-ill child I had just examined, admitted, and started on treatment. It was four-thirty am. I cannot recall, no matter how I have tried over the years, anything of the hours or transitions in-between, though I can still remember every charted detail, down to the name, of the child I admitted that night. He had a septic joint, right hip, and he survived without residual defect.

I got it right and I know, even today, more than four decades later, that if I need to I can rise fully awake and be ready to do whatever has to be done at the first ring of the telephone. But that anecdote, which illustrates part of the conditioning of medical training in the early 1960s, does not describe good medicine, nor good patient care.

We "learned on" patients, especially poor patients, in ways that are not sanctioned today. The general rule of your progress was, in the cynical parlance of young doctors-in-training, "See one, Do one, Teach one." There was always somebody a rung or so up the ladder for you to call, but you were much more on your own than is the case today.

My point is not to assert that it was "better," or that we were somehow "stronger" than today's young doctors. That is nonsense. But medicine was, even that short time ago, much less science-based, much less super-sub-specialized, much less technology-driven, much less dependent on sophisticated laboratory and imaging guidance. It was just different, that's all. But I think it encouraged a more independent and tough-minded development, and for the many of us who were omnivorous and with insatiable appetites, there was plenty to feed on.

One might also say that the then-system also encouraged a narrowness of perspective, a neglect of life's other dimensions, and an arrogance of intellect. Perhaps so.

I had drawn, or been assigned, what seemed to be the unlucky short scheduling straw, and my two-weeks' annual vacation came after only the first six weeks of my internship, which had begun in July. This was a vacation coming long before I needed or wanted it. At that stage, I was afraid I might MISS something! But I used the opportunity to explore what turned out to be the specific map for the road to Kathmandu.

One of the Selective Service options for young physicians in that peace-time but Cold War environment, albeit an environment where just about everybody, eventually, did their two years, was an odd-and somewhat little-noticed one. John Kennedy's Peace Corps needed staff physicians overseas. If you and the Peace Corps came to agreement, they had an arrangement whereby you then received a Commission in the U.S. Public Health Service, with automatic assignment to the Peace Corps, and got your two-year Selective Service obligation fulfilled in the process. It sure sounded good to me, and beat the prospect of possibly spending two years doing induction physicals on healthy young recruits at Fort Leonard Wood, Missouri. Besides, it was a guaranteed way of getting overseas into the environment that I had already decided I was seeking.

So, without telling anyone at the hospital, I filled out and sent in an endless series of application forms, and made an appointment to go down to Washington during the first week of my August vacation and see what might happen.

The original Peace Corps headquarters building on lower Connecticut Avenue, directly across Lafayette Park from the White House, was a buzzing hive of energy and enthusiasm. When the receptionist said, "We have interviews scheduled for you with several regional directors and desk officers, Dr. Joseph." I turned and looked behind me, wondering who she was talking to. Back in Boston, as a beginning intern, I was more used to being addressed as, "Hey, You." Or sometimes, "Hold onto that." Or most usually, "You think WHAT?"

I had meetings with several gung-ho types, most of them a bit long in the tooth but with a gleam in their eye. Some appeared to be former OSS people left over from World War Two, still looking for adventure, and that was okay in my book. I was looking for adventure too.

"Well, Dr. Joseph, we have a spot opening up in Sarawak-Sabah. Lot of tropical diseases, Sea Dyaks, head-hunters, that sort of thing. Interested?"

Thanks but no thanks. Jungles aren't so much my thing as mountains.

"We need a second or third doctor in Iran. Probably base him or her in the far south, along the Persian Gulf, at the new oil refinery city of Abadan. I was there, (wink) with the Brits during the Big Show, don't you know. How does that sound?"

About as interesting as Houston, Texas, Old Chappie. Besides, I want my OWN country.

"Doctor Joseph, as Peace Corps' Regional Director for West Africa, I must tell you that your spoken French is atrocious. But maybe we could use you."

Pardonnez-moi, m'sieur, but didn't you say your name was Manchewiecz?

"Yes, we are planning to help the Afghans start a new medical school at Jalalabad, just at the foot of the Khyber Pass. But I must say, frankly, Dr. Joseph, that we have in mind several other physicians with quite a bit more experience and relevant credentials than you have. Sorry."

And then, just before lunchtime, a desk officer said, "Well, we do need someone to be the solo doctor in Nepal. Might that interest you?"

Bingo. I wasn't sure exactly where Nepal was, or what was in it, except for Mount Everest. And I sort of had it confused with Shangri-La, which wasn't completely off the mark. And so I said, "Well, perhaps it might. Let's talk seriously about it after lunch." I then ran off to the National Geographic Society building and library, just a few blocks away, and looked up everything they had on Nepal, beginning with "N."

At our meeting after lunch I demonstrated my encyclopedic knowledge and interest in the mountain kingdom of Nepal, and was told, "You seem to know quite a bit about Nepal. It might be a good fit. We'll let you know."

In those early days, believe it or not, Sargent Shriver, the first Director of the Peace Corps, himself President Kennedy's brother-in-law, personally interviewed every serious candidate for an overseas staff position, including the doctors. He was my last scheduled appointment for the day, at about four pm.

When I got to his office, my brain still feverish with visions of the Himalayas, his secretary said, "Dr. Joseph, Mr. Shriver's plane has been detained in Boston. He knows he has an appointment with you, and has instructed me to tell you that if you can wait, perhaps for several hours, he will definitely come to the office to see you, as soon as his plane gets him in."

It was uncharitable of me, but I thought that this was perhaps a polite way to brush off an unimportant visitor. I said to the secretary, "Are you sure that Mr. Shriver will be coming back. Maybe . . .

"Dr. Joseph," she replied frostily, "Mr. Shriver always keeps his appointments. Always." And, with more than a hint of irritation, she turned back to her electric typewriter.

His secretary was long gone, and it was after six-thirty in the evening, when Sarge Shriver blew into the office, threw his hat at the rack (he missed), and without turning his head and looking at me, said, "Hi, Steve Joseph, right? Give me a minute to get settled, Doctor, and then let's have a talk."

We shot the breeze for more than an hour and a half, over several fingers of Scotch: about Peace Corps, about Nepal, which he had recently visited, and about Boston. That's the way Sarge was, and the energy of spirit that he communicated, and that's the way the Peace Corps operated in those beginning years. By the end of the "interview" you couldn't have kept me away from that job with wild horses, if they would have me.

Well, as you already know, they took me. The internship year flew by. I was on duty on the acute-care wards during the November weekend of the assassination of JFK. I have confused and bizarre memories of going from room to room about my work, seeing montage slices on the televisions over the beds, of Oswald, Jack Ruby, the funeral cortege, the white horse with the boots reversed in the stirrups, John-John's salute, and the rest.

I tried, as best I could, to prepare myself for what would be, on the one hand, a general practice plus the opportunity for "tropical pediatrics," and, on the other, an unusual environment and a range of pathology that I didn't learn much about in medical school.

I spent extra time in the surgical emergency room, trying to gain dexterity and judgement in minor surgical procedures. I had some friends among the interns in the pediatric dentistry program, and they gave me an informal crash course, during the wee hours, when the senior people were not around, in dental local anesthesia and extractions but not in filling teeth, just pulling them. They presented me with a short set of dental extraction forceps, obviously purloined, but who was asking? These later served their purpose in the far hills of Nepal on a number of occasions. I tried to learn as much acute infectious disease as possible, and concentrated on the bread and butter stuff rather than on the abstruse and academic.

When, back in September, I learned that the Public Health Service would offer me a Commission, and that Peace Corps would take me and assign me as the solo doctor in Nepal, I had to go see my Chief of Medicine and tell him that I would not be staying on for the next year. I explained to him what I wanted to do, and, not very clearly, because I wasn't very clear myself, why I wanted to do it.

In those days, hierarchical relationships were pretty formal in teaching hospitals, and authority structures were rigidly maintained, especially in Boston. Teaching hospital residencies were "pyramidal," which meant that on each yearly rung of the ladder, there were fewer positions than on the rung below. It was unusual to take some time out and then come back, you usually just had to look for somewhere else. Believe it or not, we all stood up when the attending or senior physician, or even the chief resident, came onto the ward or into the room. Thus, I approached the meeting with the Chief of Medicine with trepidation.

Dr. Janeway (I still, forty years later, and after years of further interaction, can never think of him as "Charlie," though I loved and respected him dearly) peered at me through his beetled bushy snow-white eyebrows. I knew that he had sowed a few wild oats of his own in Iran as a young doctor before taking up a distinguished research and academic career, and that he still maintained an active interest in the pediatrics of what was then called the "developing world."

"Steve," he said. "You go do what you want to do, and give it your best in learning and doing. When you're ready to come back, let me know. There will be a place here for you." And that was that.

In the spring, Peace Corps arranged for some evening tutoring in

Nepali. They dug up a Bengali over in Cambridge who supposedly spoke the language. I had trouble keeping my eyes open, but by June I could at least do *"eck,dui,din,char,panch" and "Namaste!"* I read all I could find about Nepal, about the Gurkhas, geography, sociology, anthropology, current history, anything I could get my hands on. Once or twice, half-asleep for morning rounds after a hard night on call, I even answered in ungrammatical Nepali when asked a medical question by the chief resident. I guess I was the pretty odd duck I appeared to be, but I was doing what I wanted most to be doing in all the world: being an intern, and preparing to go off to another set of Shining Mountains.

July first rolled around; my intern-mates, newly anointed as junior assistant residents, probably hardly noticed that I was gone. Gathering in Washington, the fifty or so of us who were shipping out to various countries around the globe had a ten-day Public Health Service and Peace Corps medical orientations. I met some people who have become life-long friends, and dozed through the administrative bumpf. Then half of us, those who were slated for Africa, the Middle East, and Asia, went up to New York for a two-week crash course at Columbia University in tropical medicine. The other half, assigned to Latin America or the Pacific, went down to Tulane in New Orleans for an analogous program. I learned to recognize all the bad little wiggly things that can be found in your blood, stool, or urine, and how, at least, to find my way around the standard textbooks of tropical medicine to plan diagnosis and treatment.

And then it was time to go. Departure via Pan Am from New York set for August 9. On the morning of August 8, 1964, we heard confused radio bulletins of an attack on U.S. naval vessels in some far-off place called the Gulf of Tonkin. What did it mean? Departure postponed? Change in assignments? No. Go. And off we went.

3

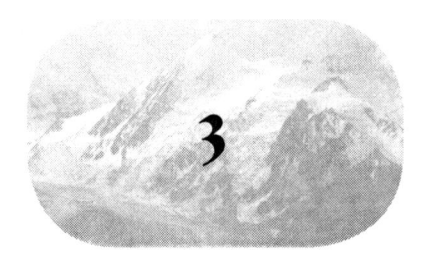

Once I realized that "I wasn't in Boston anymore," it was clear to me that I had a great deal of learning to do, across a wide variety of fronts. I needed to make myself as competent as possible in the basic skills of diagnosis and management of the health problems that might appear in both Westerners and Nepalis. But I also needed to gain some expertise in the intricate logistics of getting from one place to another, and communicating with my patients about this. Further, I needed to understand the way the trail system could be made to work for or against me. I would need to understand the physical and psychological characteristics of the volunteers, individually as patients, and collectively as a population. And, finally, I would need to work out the best possible system by which the far-flung PCVs in this virtually-roadless country could engage in as much self-care as possible, both preventive (safe trekking habits such as, for example, not traveling by night), and therapeutic (such as how to best recognize and treat simple diarrhea). I realized that, far from coming out to Nepal as "The Doctor" who was well equipped to solve all problems, my education was just commencing.

Gobbling up information on diagnosis and treatment was something I had a lot of experience doing. I had had a solid basic medical education, but only one year of practical experience as an intern. I knew how to use the books in the small but well-chosen medical library the Peace Corps provided. Of special pleasure among them was the venerable 'Manson's *Tropical Diseases*' which I pored over until the pages came loose and the hard blue cover turned grimy. This was a labor of love, for Manson, a traditional British medical text, is filled with the anecdotes and trivia of the discoveries and adventures of the early European medical pioneers, often military physicians, in Africa and Asia, with a lesser-focus on Latin America. It had wonderful colored plates, many of them hand-drawn in the old-style, and enough photographs of the more horrific and spectacular tropical and parasitic maladies to keep me from falling asleep over its pages.

A larger problem was who to ask for general knowledge and specific advice. This relative lack of easy access to authoritative teachers was, for me, the main source of my sense of medical isolation, much more acute than not having someone at my elbow to guide decision-making in any particular case. I had the American surgeon at Shanta Bhawan, my friend Keith in Banepa, and Florence out at USAID; beyond that there wasn't much. I was too isolated in Nepal to have much contact with Peace Corps doctors in other countries, except for a worldwide newsletter, circulated monthly, and a once-yearly regional meeting that lasted for several days. Mail was unreliable, medical journals arrived sporadically. I could, of course, always get rapid consultative help by cable from specialists arranged through Peace Corps/Washington for a specific individual's problem. What I couldn't get, and missed most, was the context of on-going learning and discussion that had been a central element in shaping my life for the past nine years, through university, medical school, and internship. So I studied hard, thought long, and looked to my patients to teach me.

I tried to break my communications and logistical issues into some rational schema. For communications, it was telephone within Kathmandu, and nowhere else. I have already described the monthly mailgrams and the wireless telegram system. It then occurred to me that I should reverse the process as well, and that I should write a newsletter that would be sent to all the PCVs monthly, going out with their other mail and received whenever the erratic mail service allowed. In it I tried not to sound too didactic or preachy about how to stay healthy and what to do when you're not, but I am not sure, given the ways of young doctors, that I succeeded.

I soon realized there was no substitute for getting out and spending time on site with the volunteers, who were much hungrier for a fresh face to sit around and pass the evening hours in conversation with than they were for another communiqué from Kathmandu. I made it a practice to do as much routine visiting as possible. That meant that I spent about a third of all my time in Nepal out on the trails, staying with volunteers in their village homes, placing more emphasis on health education and disease prevention than on the episodes of illness.

This was a two-edged sword, of course, as I had learned on my first trek. If I wasn't sitting around the firehouse in Kathmandu waiting for the alarm bell to ring, I was more liable to not be there when it did. And that realization, of course, brought me back to an emphasis on logistics.

For routine travel, I could fly commercially to six or seven key locations in the country, and then walk a circuit, usually of a week or ten days, stopping at the volunteers' villages en route, before taking another flight back to Kathmandu. Ten days is a long time to be away from the fire alarm, and this was a constant source of worry, but it seemed about the best mix of doing my job both "out there" and in Kathmandu. There was nowhere that I could travel by motor vehicle, except within the Kathmandu Valley, and on the short spur roads that led from the southern Terai airfields to the start of the foot trails I trekked along up into the hills.

For emergencies, assuming the communications part of it worked, I was much better placed. The Embassy had a fixed-wing STOL (short take-off and landing) aircraft that could land on the shortest grass airstrip, and also a three seater helicopter, four seats, if you had to strap a litter onto the side in a pinch. Peace Corps could rent time, but the cost was very expensive for the modest Peace Corps budget. I tried to minimize use of these aircraft to when I truly needed them, especially for the helicopter, which of course could fly and land anywhere, right into the middle of a tiny and isolated village, usually landing on the schoolyard or soccer field.

I soon realized, however, that if I said I needed urgent air transport, Willi would never deny me access to it. How could he? I began to develop an intricate system of maximizing the efficiency of getting from here to there and back. If I had to go from point A to point C on a suspected emergency, and the life or death threat turned out to be a false alarm, with no necessity to evacuate the PCV by helicopter back to Kathmandu for observation or treatment, there was no reason why I couldn't just drop into point B in-between, just to make a routine visit and see that everything was all right.

The volunteers, every one of them, hated this practice, as it turned their whole village upside down for days. Imagine if you had never seen a road, or a motor car, or a washing machine, or any energized devices except for a flashlight and a battery-powered crackly old radio. Then, without warning, this shiny whirlybird buzzes the village and drops out of the sky, right on top of your kids' soccer match, swirling dust up into the sky from the dirt field so you can't see as well as can't hear. Out jumps a Westerner with a big bag, off he goes to the Peace Corps house, can't stop to take care of anyone else because time is literally money, and lots of it. The pilot stays with the bird for the half-hour it is on the ground, trying to hold back the crowd who want to touch it and climb all over it. Then the two of them jump back into the helicopter and rise into the sky with more dust and more noise, and are gone as abruptly as they came. Now, if you were the PCV teaching English to primary school children in that village, in a one-room, thatched-roof, mud-walled schoolhouse with precious few books and no audio-visual aids, how could you explain what had just gone on, or why it was useful? I could see the volunteers' point of view on this, but I also tried to use every opportunity I could get to "visit" with them.

I also must admit it was great fun to ride that chopper, flying along the highest mountains in the world, sitting in a Plexiglas bubble. And it did give me tremendous capability to answer the bell, provided I knew it had rung.

This infinitely complex dance of logistics sometimes held real surprises. One day, I received a three-day old telegram in Kathmandu, relayed by runner from a site where we had two bridge-builders in an extremely remote work location in the jungle *Terai*, camped alongside the river they were bridging, a day's walk from the nearest town and wireless site.

SEVERE TOOTH PAIN THREE DAYS STOP FACE SWOLLEN COME QUICK END.

Damn. The usual problem of uncertainty. Is this just dental caries? More likely, it sounds like a dental abscess. Almost a week now, since symptoms began. This could prove serious trouble. Should we crank up the chopper, grab the forceps and everything else and go? Now? Yep. No choice.

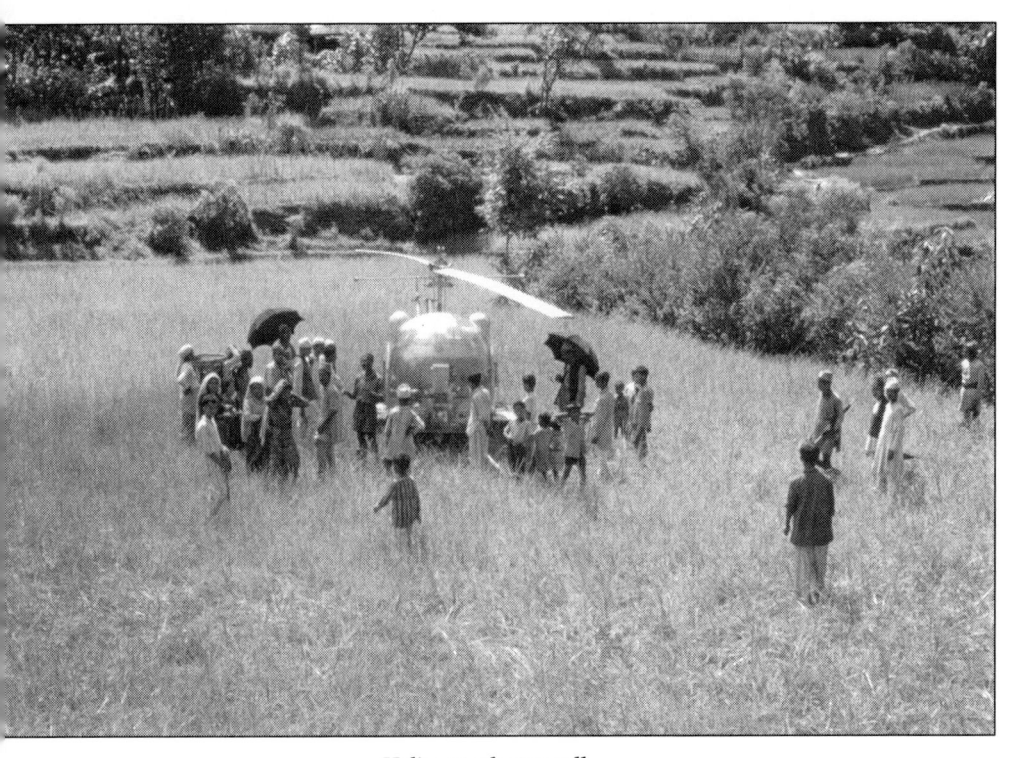

Helicopter house call

Ernie, the helicopter pilot, was, like his pilot partner, an ex-Air America contractor in Vietnam and elsewhere in Southeast Asia. You didn't want to know what cargoes they had been flying, or for whom. He found the remote site, with some difficulty, about forty minutes' flight from Kathmandu, or a week's walk if there was any way to walk it. As we circled and descended into the riverside clearing, there, among a group of Nepali co-workers, stood our two PCVs. One was smiling and waving—but wait, as we got closer I could see that the smiling waving one was the supposed dental emergency.

As we landed, he ducked under the slowing blades, rushed up to the chopper and said, "I'm all right now, Doc, guess it was just a toothache. That oil of cloves in my medical kit really worked. But, anyway, thanks for coming."

Before I told him that I had better just take a look anyway, since we had spent about a thousand dollars getting me to him, I cast a glance at the *other* volunteer. He was standing quietly and unsteadily, his skin and eyeballs as yellow as the noon-day sun, and, as luck would have it, while I was getting out of the helicopter he began to have a shaking chill.

It took about ten seconds to make the diagnosis of malaria, for which the T*erai* was infamous, and to throw him, shaking away, into the chopper's third seat. The other guy we had to leave where he was, with his toothache, and hope that the oil of cloves would keep it at bay until he could walk out to the Indian border and make his way by air or road to Kathmandu and the Mission Hospital dentist's foot-powered drill.

By the time I got him back to my office, the "wrong guy" had finished with nearly shaking apart the helicopter, and had spiked his fever to 105 degrees I got him started on treatment, spent an hour making blood smears and staining them for malaria, put him in my house, and he pulled through just fine. Seems the two of them didn't like to take their bitter antimalarial prophylaxis. Apart from wondering why he was turning yellow, he thought the early days of chills and fever were nothing special. That helicopter, with no thanks to me or my patient, may well have saved his life. The thanks go to the guy who sent the false alarm.

There were quite a few false alarms like that. The Israeli Embassy received a week-old telegram from Jomosom, up near the Tibetan border.

HELP QUICK LEG BROKEN END.

They knew that there was a lone trekking Israeli tourist up there. Or maybe, I wondered later, could he have been an intelligence agent, spying along the frontier?

The Israeli Ambassador contracted for the U.S. helicopter and asked me to go up and get him out. It is a long way to Jomosom, and involves some beautiful flying past the Annapurna Range and up the gorge of the Kali Ghandaki into which we had to set down because of a sudden hail squall. When we got up to Jomosom, there was our patient, nursing a mildly twisted ankle. He could have waited five days and then walked out. I was all for leaving him there, though I had enjoyed the ride immensely, but his embassy had paid about five thousand dollars for the trip, so we brought him in. Definitive treatment consisted of an ACE bandage, which he had in his pack.

They weren't all false alarms, and I picked up my share of dysenteries, pneumonias, a severe depression or two, and a couple of nasty infected pilonidal cysts. Most often, the most difficult part of the entire medical diagnostic and management process was at the very start: trying to decide whether or not to crank up the bird.

In the course of those two years, I learned a great deal about the hand crafted Nepali trail system. The major routes were surprisingly well built and maintained, the result of centuries of development and use. You would find well-laid stone staircases on steep pitches out in the middle of nowhere. Rock cliffs along steep river gorges would have been hacked out, and in later years, dynamited, to form hanging trails high above the river.

One of the most beautiful features along the Nepali trails were the *chautaras*, stone walls forming a rectangle around packed earth. These were constructed over the course of centuries as resting places for travelers, especially porters. The stone walls, usually two-stepped, were sized so that a porter, carrying his load on a tumpline, could lean back and rest, still standing, against the wall with the weight of his load set on the lower level of the *chautara*. The *chautaras*, often placed at the culmination of a long, hard, hill climb, were always shady, and this was associated with their most lovely characteristic: In the earthen center surrounded by the structure, two trees were traditionally planted, and these eventually grew to huge size in the climate of the hills. One was a *pipal* (fig) tree, and one was a *bhodi* (banyan). To the Hindus, the intertwined union of *bhodi* and *pipal* symbolized the union of the god Shiva and his consort Parbati. And to the Buddhists, the *bhodi* is the tree under which the Buddha sat and received enlightenment.

After a long, dry, hot climb up the ridge, all were welcome to rest at the *chautara*. I could settle my pack and lean back, a few feet from a group of smiling Tamang or Gurung or Rai porters. We would gossip and joke with one another as best we could, in broken Nepali or fractured English.

"Ah, Bhai (Younger Brother), these hills get steeper and longer every year!"

"Yes, my friend, but the mountains stay as beautiful as ever, just like the young Gurung girls."

"That is true, but to be a poor porter is a hard life. Here, take a cigarette, Bhai."

And the breeze would blow softly through the *bhodi* and *pipal,* the birds, attracted to the fruit, would sing, and I would feel the everlasting sweetness of the hills.

There was almost never snow on the trails in the hills, not below about 10,000 feet. Most of the year there was water aplenty from springs, often nearby to a *chautara*, or from small streams, though you always had to treat the water as heavily contaminated, and had to watch out that you didn't get water leeches into the rim of your canteen, or, worst of all, from there on up your nose. Monsoon rains would make the trails, especially in the lower and more level elevations, muddy and slippery.

But some ridge climbs could be hot and dry and seemingly endless. The volunteers had a good system for grading climbs when describing routes to others. There was a particularly long and steep ridge to climb in the east, going from Dharan up to the village of Dhankuta. As you came out of a dry riverbed and started up, the climb itself took just about two hours, with scarcely a leveling out along the way. Volunteers would describe other ridge climbs in comparative values: a "two-Dhankuta," or a "one-Dhankuta" ridge.

Just at the base of the Dhakuta climb, in a dusty farmyard on the far side of the streambed, I was transfixed by the sight of he whom I came to call Howling Man, or even Beast Man. He was all skin and bone, filthy, and ragged. His left leg was held by a strong chain that was fastened to a stout post in the middle of the yard. Worn into the dirt were grooves from his constant and aimless circling of the post.

When he saw me, he howled and raged, and leaped so hard to the end of his chain that he was thrown bodily to the ground, like a ferocious dog at the end of that chain, only to rise again and again, to howl and try to break free. I knew that, should that chain give way, any passerby would likely be torn to pieces.

I saw Howling Man three or four times on journeys up to Dhankuta, which is a central point for travel elsewhere in the eastern hills. He was always the same, and I never saw another person in the farmhouse or in the yard. And then, one time I passed by, and he was not there. The house behind the post sat empty and silent. The post remained, but not the chain, and I never saw him again.

River crossings could be anything from splashing across to cool your boots to truly terrifying ordeals. Across some of the smaller rivers the "bridge" consisted of simply three thick ropes: one to balance your feet on and two higher ones for handholds as you shuffled across. Then there were all manner of wood plank and rope guideline bridges.

At nearly a score of strategic locations across major rivers in the hills, you would come across a quite astonishing sight: stone- and iron- towered foot bridges with thick steel cables, strung in a modern suspension style. Two additional steel cables formed the supports for the wooden planking of the bridge itself, though often individual planks or sections of planking were rotted or missing; you had to be careful. Metal placards on the bridge towers proclaimed: "Edinborough Iron Works, 1933." Apparently, in the 1930s, these bridges were built by the British, and had remained as the major transportation links on the trails up through the present time.

But the worst way to cross wide Nepali rivers was by ferry or dugout canoe, and these were usually to be found on the largest and swiftest rivers. A plank boat or a dugout would be drawn across the current attached to a guide wire. Or, worst of all, a long dugout, full of porters and their loads, and the occasional Peace Corps trekker, would simply be set on a diagonal course across the current, with a paddler in bow and stern. Each time I crossed a river this way, I was relieved when we only crashed into the opposite bank. One waited for the tippy dugout to overturn, overloaded with gear and with porters, most of whom could not swim.

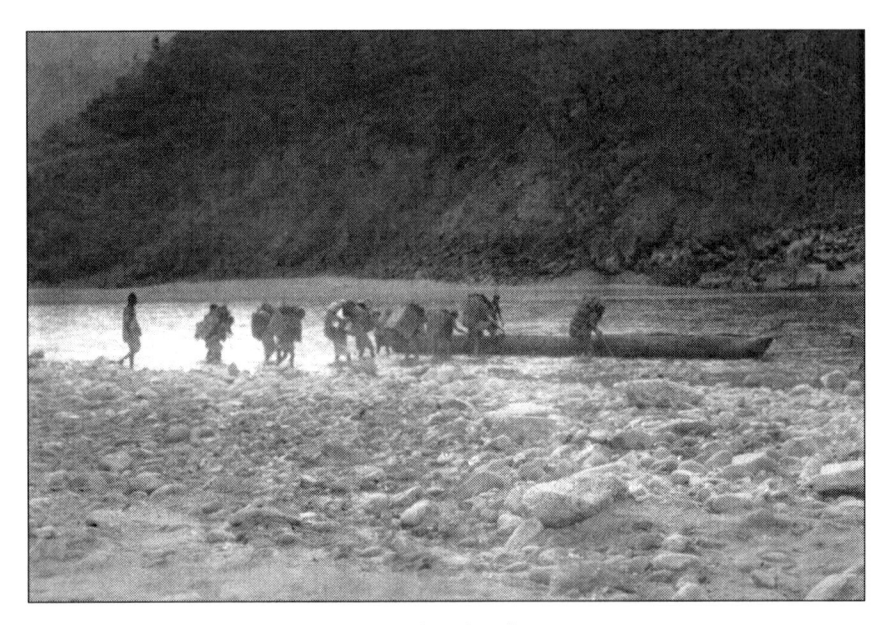

Porters crossing river by canoe

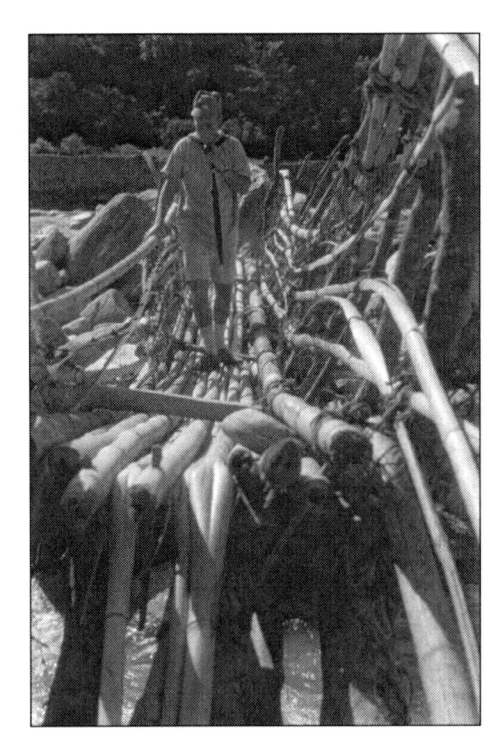

Volunteer crossing bamboo bridge

One afternoon, I received the proverbial end-of-day telegram from a volunteer in Dhankuta:

SICKBAD POX STOP COME FAST END.

What could it signify? Smallpox still existed in the hills, but all PCVs were vaccinated before coming to Nepal. Chickenpox was ever-present, especially at this season, but most Americans had chickenpox in childhood. Perhaps it wasn't really a pox disease. Or perhaps it was a case of chickenpox in a volunteer who had escaped the childhood disease (there was, at that time, no vaccine against chickenpox). In that case, there was little to fear of a truly urgent nature, though chickenpox can be a more severe disease in adults. In the worst case, perhaps the volunteer had had an ineffective smallpox vaccination, and in truth was suffering from smallpox in a village outbreak that we hadn't heard about yet. This would truly pose an emergency.

I couldn't really judge the situation from Kathmandu. Should I wait for further information, which might not be forthcoming? The telegram was four days old already. Should I go immediately? Wait for morning?

It was already almost mid-afternoon, and there were no more flights to Biratnagar, the town on the Indian border from which I could get a jeep to Dharan, and then start the 4- or 5-hour walk up to Dhankuta.

I checked the volunteer's medical file. He had been vaccinated against smallpox in 1963, a vaccination good for at least ten years—IF a positive take had ensued. I could find nothing in his history about chickenpox or no-chickenpox. What to do? Always the arch-conservative, I threw my pack together (15 minutes), arranged for the Embassy STOL to fly me to Biratnagar (15 minutes of discussion), drove to the airstrip (20 minutes), and we were airborne 15 minutes later for the hour-and-a-half flight.

I grabbed a Jeep taxi for the 20 mile trip to Dharan, at the base of the hills, and was knocking at the door of the PCV house in Dharan bazaar just as dusk settled. The volunteers fed me a quick cold meal as I explained the situation to them. They did not let me off lightly for my past exhortations that trekking at night was dangerous and should never be undertaken. I humped my load and moved off, ten miles or more to cover that night.

Fortunately, there was a good early moon in a clear sky and I did not need to make much use of the flashlight. The first couple of hours went smoothly, save for anxiety about the village dogs, who barked threateningly and followed me into the darkness as I passed through several small settlements. On the crest of the first small ridge, before you descend to the dry riverbed and then start the long climb of "one-Dhankuta," I stopped at a teahouse. A few villagers sat around a small fire.

"Where are you going, Sahib? You have a heavy pack and the trails are dangerous in the dark. There are still tigers in these hills, roaming at night. One should not travel in the dark. We have heard the tiger near here, and do not go out at night."

I told myself that they were pulling my leg, and better them than the tiger. I almost gave in to myself and stopped for the night in the teahouse, thinking I could start up again at first light. Then I got stubborn, and resolved to press on.

Well, the tiger didn't get me, if indeed there was a tiger within a hundred miles of the trail. But I sweated every step, and froze at every strange sound, and I hope my teahouse companions had a good laugh at my expense. At least I hope that was the case, better a practical joke than sound advice not heeded.

A bit before midnight, I was banging on the door of the volunteers' house in Dhankuta. The telegram-sender answered the door, rubbing his eyes, wakened from a peaceful sleep, naked to the waist. His trunk bore the unmistakable pustules and scabs of centrally located lesions in all different stages of development: chickenpox, and certainly not smallpox. "Yeah, I guess I got it from my kids at school. There's been a lot of it going around. It was pretty itchy, but I'm on the mend now. Let me make you a cup of tea, since you've come all this way."

I rolled my bag out on his floor, slept well, and we had a good laugh about it in the morning. "Skin to skin," so to speak, from Kathmandu to the top of "one-Dhankuta" in under ten hours, and I had even remembered to bring the mail.

All the traveling I did gave me plenty of opportunity to hold impromptu village clinics, and this I found one of the most enjoyable parts of my job. I would set up shop in the volunteers' house, or at the local school, or under a shady tree on the *tundikhel* (village square or playing field). Sometimes a few patients, or even a single individual, would show up, sometimes many would come. I saw many conditions that I could do nothing about, and many where I could offer only symptomatic treatment, but I also could sometimes make a real difference.

Under the trees in a small village three days' distance from Pokhara's excellent mission hospital, a mother held up a child of perhaps two years old. The child was wasted, almost skeletal. His breathing came in short sharp gasps, and the flesh between his ribs pulled inward with each breath. A dry, paroxysmal, non-productive cough took most of his energy. His color was gray, and his skin clammy but feverish. His eyes were dull, and the skin around his lips was dry and cracked. Snapping, crackling, and whistling sounds came into my stethoscope, especially from the upper front portions of his chest.

"He has been sick for four months, Doctor Sahib. He coughs and coughs, just like his father at home has done for two years now."

I was quite sure that the child was dying of tuberculosis, like so many others in the hills of Nepal. I told, and then begged, the mother to carry the child to Pokhara and the Shining Hospital.

"How can I go?" she said. "I have three other children at home, and my man has been sick for a long time. It is a far way to Pokhara. Who will make rice and care for my family if I go? Who will cultivate our paddy? This child will be taken from me anyway, as two have before him. No, I must stay here. Cannot you give him some medicine to take the sickness away? Give me some, please, Doctor Sahib."

Allowing myself the ridiculous illusion that there was a slight chance that this was a simple acute pneumonia, I gave the child a large injection of penicillin and some follow-up tablets. I knew that none of this would do anything against the tuberculosis. The child would surely die. I felt a fraud, sheltering myself from the mother's plaintive grief with what amounted to a quack's nostrum.

But some patients would go to the hospital, no matter how far off it was. Once, trekking the gorge of the Arun Khola beyond Chainpur in eastern Nepal, I came upon a porter carrying a heavy load along the narrow cliffside trail. It was a huge woven basket, with the rear side cut out so that the basket made a kind of rattan chair, protected from the sun and rain by the basket's top. In the chair slumped an old man, skin and bones, wasted so that all you really focused on were the deep-socketed eyes. Cancer? Tuberculosis? The porter, supporting his load on a tumpline, could hardly raise his head as we passed each other. He mumbled "*Namaste,*" and shuffled on silently down the trail. I turned and watched the skeletal old man's eyes until they disappeared around the next bend.

But sometimes you could make a real difference, and sometimes in strange ways.

Up in the Solo Khumbu, the impossibly-lovely Sherpa region that is the gateway to Sagarmatha, which we call Everest, and the Tibetans call Chomolungma, they brought a boy of about nine years to see me. His right arm was splinted straight out, and wrapped in filthy rags. Four or five weeks earlier, he had injured, fractured as it turned out, his elbow in a fall. Someone, I never learned who, had splinted the arm straight out, and left it that way. Now the fracture was mostly healed, and the boy had a straight stick for a right arm.

Take your right arm and hold it unbent, straight out. Now try and scratch your nose, or bring food to your mouth, or do a hundred other things that you must do each day, especially if you are a yak-herder and potato farmer in the Solo Khumbu.

Two things I had learned in Boston came to mind: Never deal with an elbow fracture in a child, before the growth plates have fused, without an x-ray. Never leave an arm to heal in an unflexed position. And I also remembered the cardinal rule of medicine: "First, do no harm."

But the nearest x-ray was an impossible week or more away. And the boy's arm was locked straight. So, harm or not, I re-broke it. I heard the collective sharp intake of breath from the small crowd around us as I did it.

I had some injectable anesthetic in my bag, and a few rolls of dry plaster. He made no sound when I slid in the local anesthetic, nor when I snapped the stick of his arm into a right angle bend. Tough little Sherpa kid, he just squeezed his eyelids tight over a few tears. I soaked the plaster in a wooden bucket, and put it on to dry as two halves of a somewhat loose cast, wrapped it snugly in gauze, and fashioned a sling. I told the parents what to watch for with the cast, and when to remove it.

Now bend your arm into a right angle at the elbow. See all the things that you can do with that arm, using only rotation at the shoulder and wrist. You can feed and care for yourself and your family. You can use tools. You can be a farmer.

I sometimes dream about that Sherpa boy, who by now may be a grandfather. In my dream he is smiling, as Sherpas are wont to do. Sitting on his knee, encircled by that stiff but useable right arm, is his small grandson, who will also some day be a farmer.

Late in my tour in Nepal, Willi Unsoeld led a group of us on a trek up to the old Everest base camp at an altitude of 19.000 feet. This was before the days of commercial tourism. We had a few Sherpas with us, but carried our own light packs. We moved, from the new grass airstrip at Lukla, up through Namche Bazaar. We sat with the lamas of the holy monasteries. At Thyang Boche, the temple bell was fashioned from a discarded oxygen cylinder left by some mountaineering expedition, and we sat and drank buttered yak tea with the Abbot, in a room whose wooden walls were painted round with murals. At Pyang Boche, we held in our hands the scalp and skullbone said to have come from the *yeti*, the Abominable Snowman. Willi told us that the skull had been sent to the London Museum, where experts were unable to identify the species of primate it had belonged to. The Abbot of Pyang Boche just smiled and nodded. We slept in ruined roofless huts built of stone, at the cold high gray-green yak pasture of Gorak Shep, already deserted at this high altitude in mid-August. We made our highest camp on the site of Willi's Everest base camp, at the foot of the ice fall. Standing straight, with our heads tipped back as far as they could go, we could not see the top of the mountain.

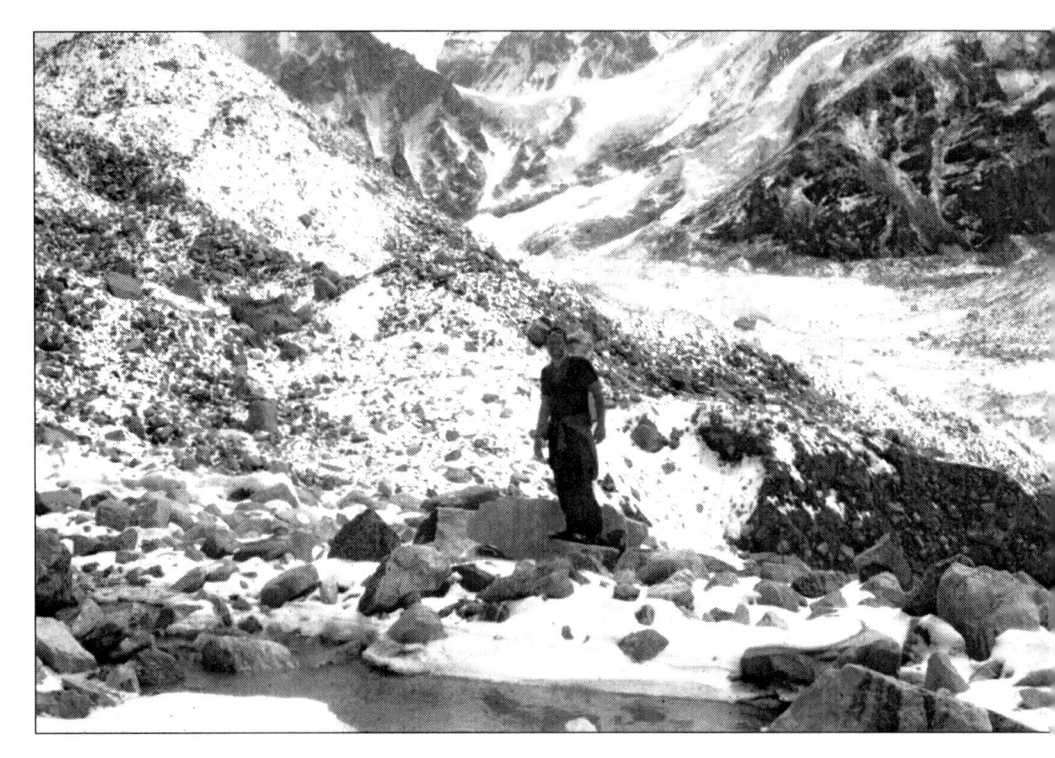

Everest Base Camp and the Ice Fall

On our way back down, we turned a bit east on a smaller trail, and passed through the Sherpa village of Kunden. Women plowed potato fields with yaks, under the looming triangular peak of Ama Dablam. A new and empty clinic stood in the little village, donated by Sir Edmund Hillary, who, along with Tensing Norgay, first stood on Sagarmatha's summit.

I thought to myself that I would return someday, and live for a time and practice medicine in Kunden, but, as is the way with many promises that you make to yourself, I never did.

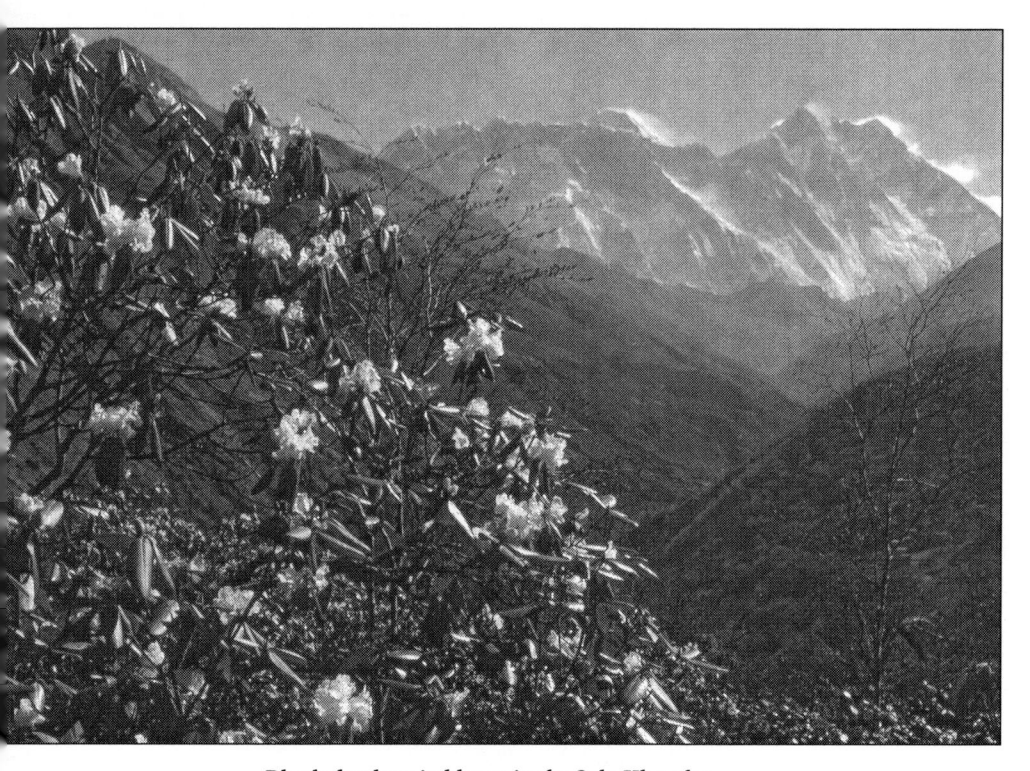

Rhododendron in bloom in the Solo Khumbu

4

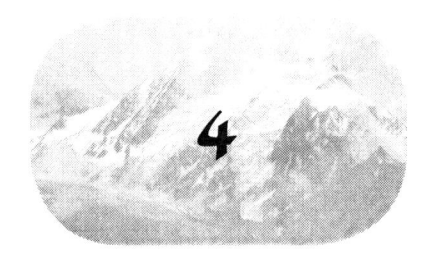

It was in the early autumn of my second year in Nepal, shortly after the monsoon rains had ended and when the high snow mountains were clearest against the newly-washed blue intensity of the sky, that I received a call on the office phone from Harry Barkely, the Embassy's Deputy Chief of Mission.

"Hi, Steve, the Ambassador would like you to drop by for a few minutes this afternoon if you could. Shall we say about three pm?"

I tried to press Harry for some idea of what it was the Ambassador wanted to discuss, but he evaded my questions. "Just come on by and we can talk about it this afternoon," he said.

"What now?" I thought to myself, not out of irritation but out of curiosity. "A junior Foreign Service officer with incipient alcoholism? A bored embassy wife caught between depression and an extramarital affair? A Marine guard with hemorrhoids or persistent diarrhea, or both? Or perhaps something I've not seen before, with larger implications for the American community here, or even some international situation. Harry isn't usually so coy. Guess we'll just have to wait and see."

The American Embassy, a featureless whitewashed three-story stucco building along the King's Road, was only a half-mile from the Peace Corps office. I parked my little blue Jeep against the curb, out of the way of the bicycle rickshaws and the occasional motor car, and the even-more occasional wandering sacred cow. I said hi to the Marine guard on duty inside the embassy entrance, and climbed the stairs to the Ambassador's office. I asked the Ambassador's secretary how the new cream I had given her for her persistent skin rash was doing, and she waved me on in.

Harry, sitting relaxed with his long legs crossed in a soft chair, dressed in gray flannel slacks and a blue blazer (not exactly the Nepalese national costume), cocked his fingers in a casual hello. Harry was, I knew, intense Yankee at the core. But he always conveyed, deliberately or not, a sort of British insouciance, borrowed straight from a novel by Evelyn Waugh. One always expected that his first words would be, "Cup of tea, old Chap?"

Ambassador Horace Stubblefield, clad as usual in a black suit, white shirt and narrow monochrome necktie, was a portly man in early middle-age, universally regarded as fair and friendly, but with a somewhat formal air always about him. His wife, who was upper crust British by birth and upbringing, was kind at heart but I always had the sense that she regarded her husband's charges, the American community, as "those troublesome Colonials." I never felt fully relaxed with either of them, though they were, as my occasional patients, pretty much the same with their pants off as the rest of us lesser mortals.

"Thank you for coming by, Steve," the Ambassador said as we shook hands. "I want to ask for your help on a matter of some importance to the embassy."

From my past experience, those words signified to me that there was an issue of considerable medical and social delicacy to discuss in confidence, usually crossing a blurred boundary between a personal medical problem and an administrative, political, or diplomatic one. I became aware, out of the corner of my eye, that a third person was standing in the office, having been partially out of sight as I pushed open the door.

Ambassador Stubblefield nodded in his direction and made the introductions. "Major Thompson, this is Dr. Steve Joseph, the Peace Corps doctor we have been speaking about. Steve, this is Bill Thompson, who flew in from Panama, via Washington, last night."

The major was a man slightly above middle-height, lean and wiry, probably in his early forties but looking like an athlete ten years younger. He had brown hair cropped short and standing up as straight as his ramrod-spined posture. A thick but well-trimmed mustache gave a hint of individuality and self-confident assertiveness to his otherwise cut-out military appearance and bearing. His deep tan, without evidence of sunburn, indicated that he probably spent more time in the Panamanian jungle, where I knew that the Special Forces had a significant training and exercise facility, than anywhere in Washington. Though he was dressed in casual civilian clothes, chin-in, chest-out, you would never make the mistake of taking him for a visiting State Department auditor, or a Third Secretary Cookie Pusher.

We shook hands, and exchanged a few polite words. He spoke softly, with an accent that was straight from the hills of Kentucky, and it was easy to surmise his lineage as third, or perhaps fifth, generation Army, all the way.

Harry took up the ball. "No, Steve, Major Thompson has not arrived needing treatment for a case of *Dehli Belly*, though that might be your first thought. He is actually here to do some trekking in Nepal, specifically to test out a new external frame backpack that the Special Forces are considering adopting."

I gave Harry my best "who do you think fell off the turnip truck?" smile. Even a Peace Corps doctor could figure out that the U.S. Special Forces would not send a field grade officer ten thousand miles to Nepal, bordering between India and Chinese-occupied Tibet, to check out the field-worthiness of a backpack.

Harry got the message, gave his lopsided grin, and shrugged. "Specifically, he would like to trek up from Butwal to Pokhara and then perhaps northwest somewhere into the higher country up around Jomosom, probably not as far as Muktinath or Mustang, definitely not, repeat not, to within ten miles of the Tibet frontier."

So. This putative backpack now required testing on a specific trail route, and it just happened to need testing up in the north where the Tibetan guerrillas, the Khambas, had a major clandestine trade and travel route back and forth between Nepal and Tibet, and where they were alleged to re-supply for their raids against the Chinese military forces in Tibet. And we just happened to have current increased tension in the region, both between India and Pakistan, and with the Chinese and their military occupation of Tibet, and little old Nepal was squeezed four ways into the middle. Not to mention other activities in Asia, such as in Vietnam, Laos,

Cambodia, and the U.S. bases in Thailand. Guess it sure was a good time to field test new equipment. But I said nothing, and waited for the next card to be played.

"Steve," put in the Ambassador, "you do about as much trail traveling in the hills as anyone except a few of the volunteers doing bridge building or community development. We thought that perhaps you could, ah, find a good reason to run one of your medical visit circuits in that area, starting in a few days. While doing that, you could serve as a guide to Major Thompson. I've had a word with Willi, and he says you generally set your own schedule, so there is no problem from that standpoint."

I tried to think on my feet. This obviously was getting uncomfortably close to, or over, the explicit line of Peace Corps prohibition against activities connected with U.S. intelligence or military interests, but I knew that line had been stretched, had even stretched it myself, upon occasion, especially if it concerned medical assistance. On the other hand, I certainly could justify a visit to the central hills and farther north. I hadn't been in that area for awhile. Besides, this guy looked like he might be fun to travel with. I might learn a few things along the way, and I probably could be useful to him with regard to my knowledge of the country.

"Of course, Mr. Ambassador," I replied, but looking directly at Harry. "This seems straightforward, and not excessively outside my own brief. It appears that Willi, as Peace Corps Director, doesn't have a problem with it."

I thought that was a nice way to cover my own tail in case anything went wrong, which it probably would, just as Willi's comments had covered his own.

"I would be delighted to have Major Thompson's company on shall we say, a routine medical visit to several PCV stations . . . and, uh, beyond. Bill, why don't we have dinner together tonight, my house, and we can talk over logistics and do some route planning. I have some current patients I need to sort out, make sure the doctors at the mission hospital across town can cover for me and so forth, but I could be ready to leave in a couple of days, say on Friday. I guess we would need about ten or twelve days for the trip; that ought to give you plenty of opportunity to decide on the field worthiness of the new, what was it, external frame pack."

And, with his back slightly turned to the Ambassador, Bill Thompson gave me a quick wink in answer to my just-suppressed grin, and I knew I had found a good trail buddy.

The drone of the propellers of the Royal Nepal Airlines DC3 was not conducive to conversation in the lightly insulated and hard-seated passenger cabin, so I closed my eyes and dozed during most of the one-and-a-half hour flight from Kathmandu to Bharaiwa. Bill and I each had our packs in the cabin with us, and no other luggage. His pack was indeed an experimental-looking outside-frame model that appeared to me to be decidedly uncomfortable for the long haul. We were both light on spare clothing, except for a generous ration of extra socks, lacking raingear, and each of us had a light sleeping bag and ground cloth lashed to the pack.

A few snacks and field rations, a quart canteen and iodine pills for disinfecting drinking water, a Sierra Club cup that did extra duty as a cooking pot or plate, flashlight, large working knife and small Swiss Army knife, a stripped-down shaving and washing kit, a hundred feet of parachute cord, a compass, maps, and fire-making capability. These comprised pretty much the rest of the basic load for each of us.

Bill was also carrying a 35 millimeter camera and several rolls of slide film. As for me, I had in addition my full medical traveling kit, the contents of which I had worked out over the past year's experience and an obsessive-compulsive nature. It included all the antibiotics I could think of, both in oral and injectable formulations, painkillers, sedatives, and hypnotics, in both oral and injectable forms, medications for symptomatic treatment of diarrheal, parasitic, and respiratory infections, emergency and resuscitative meds for injection, injectable local anesthetics, a selection of different sizes of syringes and needles and scalpel blades, various creams and ointments, a selection of bandages, disinfectants, and bleeding control materials, a couple of rolls of dry plaster casting material, my dental forceps, and an expanded minor surgical kit for suturing and for whatever treatable trauma might come my way. Whew! All told, with a stethoscope, a small flashlight, and an oto-laryngo-ophthalmascope, it brought my usual pack weight to about 50 or 60 pounds, even with the handle cut off my toothbrush, a backpacking trick I had learned from Willi. But I had also learned that I would rather carry it all than want something and be without it.

Bharaiwa was one of a series of near-identical towns that lay, from east to west, in the Nepal Terai along the border with India, where the Gangetic Plain merges into the forest and jungle of southern Nepal. From Biratnagar in the east, on through Birganj and Bharaiwa, and to Nepalganj to the west, these towns were gateways, each connected by a Jeep road running up to another town some ten or twenty miles to the north, at the base of the hills and ridges where the walking in Nepal began.

We wasted no time in hiring a Jeep taxi at the airstrip in Bharaiwa, and making for Butwal, where several households of PCVs were stationed. I introduced Bill as a "State Department Visitor to Nepal." I had my usual talks with the Volunteers individually and collectively, shook out a few pills, etc, and spent an uneventful night, after consuming the *dal bhat* and tea that were to be our standard, if monotonous, fare for the next ten days or so.

At daybreak the next morning, we gulped some tea and dry biscuits, and started up the trail from Butwal through the Adhi Khola Gorge on our long first day's trek to Tansen. Along the *khola* (river), construction was beginning on the initial stage of what was to be the first motorable road in to Pokhara from the outside world, and which would eventually reduce four or five days of porter haulage to several hours of truck traffic. In some ways, though selfish it is true, I am glad that my own time in Nepal came before that transition, before a road network, however rudimentary, knitted the country together, and opened it to the modern world.

We left Butwal behind, and then the construction machinery in the Gorge. Thus we left "it all" behind, moving into the Middle Ages and the paddy and forest splendor of rural Nepal. Bill was a good walker. He didn't waste breath on chit-chat, tried to never take a step down when we were moving up, and looked like the pack, experimental model or not, belonged on him. I could see that he was paying close attention to a set of maps that were far better and more detailed than my own crude trail map of central Nepal, and making notes and marking features he wanted to remember. I assumed that the U.S. Army was very interested in the area to be traversed by a motorable road that would, eventually, link the plains of India to the key central Nepalese hill town of Pokhara, and up towards the Tibetan/Chinese border across the high Himalayan passes. Even today, no road can move much farther directly north from Pokhara, blocked by the majestic Annapurna massif: passage here still depends on foot and yak and pony trains.

It was a magnificent time of year to be on the trail. The monsoons were over, but not long past, and the land was verdant and the sky deep clear blue, flecked with white cotton clouds that did not threaten rain. The air was cool and dry and the watercourses plentiful, but almost free of the leeches of mid-summer. As we moved north, rhododendron trees would grow to heights of thirty feet or even taller, leafy branches now abandoned by the spring flowers with which they had been laden. The local fruits of summer: apple/pear-like *naspatis*, and the tiny mandarin orange *suntalas*, could be bought for one or two *rupees* a kilo, thrown into the top of your pack and eaten as you moved along the trail. There were many varieties of small finger-like bananas, and, once in a while, you could find a rare but supreme treat, the sweet, fresh local pineapple.

Usually, when trekking Nepal, you often must move along an east-west line, and thus constantly climb up and down the north-south-running steep ridges that form the supporting buttresses of the east-west chain of the Himalaya. This makes walking more difficult, as many of the ridges require two or three steady hours of climbing up, or what can be more difficult, climbing down, along steep and rocky trails. But in this instance, once we had accomplished the hard and switch-backed climb out of the gorge itself, we were following along, and not across, a major river course. We headed roughly northeast, and so we moved for long intervals along the spine of a ridge, with a steady but gentle incline.

Because we were on the major trade route from Bharaiwa to Pokhara, we passed frequent groups of porters humping their loads along the trail.

"These little guys are plenty tough, Bill," I said. "This is the stuff that the Gurkha soldiers are made of." And indeed they were. Seldom more than "five feet nothing" in height, browned and creased by sun and rain and almost always smiling, they carried a standard porter load of eighty-eight pounds, sometimes a load and a half for the extra few rupees. The loads were carried on a tumpline passed around their foreheads. Many porters walked with a wooden staff with a short T-head, that would just fit correctly as a prop underneath the load if they had to come to a standing stop and rest on an especially long or hard hill.

They were dressed in ragged shirts and shorts, with the all-purpose *kukri* tool shoved through a midriff sash. The *kukri*, curved knife/axe/shovel/and whatnot of the hills, came in many sizes, from the two-foot-long blade used to decapitate goats and water buffaloes at the autumn *Desai* festival, down to smaller sizes for trail and household work and firewood collection. The *kukris* were usually made from the steel of old automobile springs, with bone handles, and were carried in buffalo-hide sheaths that had extra slits in them into which were stashed miniature *kukris,* good for peeling vegetables or paring toenails. I had learned early on that a mid-sized blade made a better and more versatile trail tool than the standard American "hunting knife," and always carried one in my pack.

The porters were invariably barefoot, summer and winter, and carried on top of their loads a short rough woolen cape that served as blanket and rain or snow coat. They were reliable and honest. You could contract with a porter to deliver to you a load at such and such a village, five days hence, and he would say *"Dherai dhanyibad"* ("Thank you very much") and move on up the trail. Five days later, there he would be, load intact and untouched, smiling as you came into the village. *"Namaste, Sahib, kay gornu?Ramro cha?"* ("Hi, Boss, how's it going? Everything okay?"), and only then would he expect payment.

The porters, working as hard as mules on those endless rocky trails, would seldom spare breath to sing or whistle during the day. But at night, around the campfire, cooking their little bowls of *dal bhat,* they would stoke their short straight cylindrical pipes with *ganja*, the local potent marijuana, and sing their sweet trail songs into the surrounding darkness, and laugh and joke at old stories not known to outsiders from beyond the hills. They lived a hard life; most of them were small farmers earning a little, very little, extra cash money. They were all young men; you didn't see any old porters. As rhapsodic as are my memories of the smiling porters of the Nepali Hills, it was a brutal life.

In those days, Westerners were an uncommon sight on the trails, especially Westerners humping their own loads, and as Bill and I would pass, or be passed by, porters, they would stare at us in our sturdy boots, and frame packs, and European faces and clothes. As we passed, there would be comments, clearly humorous, and chatter would fly back and forth between them, usually in a tribal dialect. How I wished I had been able to understand what they were saying about these weird Martians encountered on the trail.

Sometimes, deep in the hills, a porter would ask me, *"Namaste, Sahib, jainu Nepal-hunu-huncha?"* ("Greetings, Sir, are you going to Nepal?"). It took me a while to understand that, to him, "Nepal" was not his country, but was the term for Kathmandu, a legendary place far away, and not directly relevant to his tribal home. I learned to answer,*"Cha, Bhai, dherai dherai tarha lai Nepal!"* ("That's it, Brother, it's very, very far to Nepal!"). And we would laugh, and wink, and move on up the trail past each other, with one last set of salutations fading away between us into the distance: *"Na-a-amaste!"* . . . *"Namasc-a-a-ar!"*

Bill and I made it to Tansen, a mid-sized town well up and into the hills, late in the afternoon. Apart from a few blisters, Bill was feeling well, and clearly enjoying this walk on the far side of the moon. Tansen had one of the few mission hospitals to be found west of Kathmandu, this one very effectively run by Americans. I went through the medical tradition of making rounds with them on some of their most interesting cases, and then we ate a simple dinner and enjoyed a long evening's talk with them, and with the pair of volunteers who had run up from the nearby village where they taught English in the primary school.

It would take us another two-and-a-half days of easy walking, and thus require spending two nights more along the trail, before reaching the outskirts of Pokhara. Since Bill was not a chatty kind of guy, and since we moved steadily and took very short breaks, with only a slightly longer one at noontime, there wasn't much chance for me to press him with the questions I was anxious to probe.

The first night after Tansen, we stayed in a village house near Walling. As we climbed the ridge towards the village, we could see on the ridgetop a figure, erect at the parade rest position, awaiting us. Coming closer, we realized that he was clad in a faded olive-green uniform, and on coming closer still, we could see the rows of decorations on his chest. As we reached the top of the ridge, he snapped to attention, with a British-style salute that fairly vibrated in the air. He bellowed, "Sah! Corporal Ram Bahadur Chetri, Sah! 48th Gurkha Infantry, Sah! Italy, Burma, Malaya, Sah! Most welcome, Sah!" He faced directly at Bill Thompson, with that instinctive way that military types have of recognizing one another. It was apparent that, seeing two Westerners working their way up the hill, he had dug out his old uniform from the trunk in the corner of his mud-and-wattle house, put it on proudly, and waited to greet us.

That evening, seated on the shaded porch of his house, Ram Bahadur Chetri told us his story. Now in his forties and late of the Queen's Ghurkas, and retired on pension and living as a farmer in the hills of Nepal. Like many of his compatriots he had come down out of the hills and enlisted in the British Army at age 16. That is to say he claimed to be 16; he had probably been nearer to 15. His face was wreathed in proud smiles as he described his service, undoubtedly carried out with boundless loyalty, eternal good humor, unequalled bravery, and unparalleled ferocity, during World War Two and in the Malayan insurgency. He had come down out of the Middle Ages, saw a good part of the world from the Mediterranean to East Asia, and, like all of his fellow Ghurkas, had left an indelible mark in the hearts of any Brits who served with him. The enlistment bonus and modest salary he had accumulated allowed him to buy a small farm and a wife back in his home village upon retirement. Thus now he waited, watching the trail rising to the ridge, for the rare days when Europeans would be seen climbing towards the village, and he could put on his uniform again. Twice a year he walked the three days down, and three days back up, to visit the military depot that the British still maintained in the Terai, his pressed uniform carefully carried on his back for putting on when he reached the base. There he picked up his pension and had his medical checkup.

There was no way that we were going to be allowed to sleep anywhere but in Corporal Chetri's house, one of the finest in the village. Over our protests, they killed a chicken, and brought out the *rakshi* (a fiery distillation of grain). We spent the better part of the night hearing tales of Gurkha combat, and the wonders that Corporal Chetri had seen, and undoubtedly performed, in the outside world. He kept pressing Bill, who turned and twisted in evading direct questions, but no mere major was really fooling Corporal Chetri. Long after midnight, we rolled out our sleeping bags on the open porch, and fell asleep with the stars in our eyes. In the morning, Mrs. Chetri pressed upon us, for the trail ahead, fruit, and cold rice wrapped in banana leaves. As we followed the trail out of the village, we could see him, this time in his ragged Nepali shirt and shorts, standing at attention, his eyes upon us until we turned a bend and were out of view.

As we turned that bend, we came upon three young boys of the village who had run out with us, and then gone on ahead, chattering like birds.

They were playing a curious game, which involved one thick stick and two thin ones, each about a foot long. One of the thin sticks was laid propped up across the thick one, somewhat like a miniature see-saw. One of the boys then took the second thin stick and smacked it down smartly over the high end of the propped-up one. The propped stick then, of course, flew up in the air, and it was the job of the other two boys to catch it before it hit the ground.

"What game is that?" Bill asked the boys.

"Sah!" they barked, coming to attention. "Sah, it is 'One-o-Cat' that we are playing at, Sah!" Shades of Empire were still resonating in Walling, where the sons of all the Corporal Chetris still kept alive this centuries-old progenitor of cricket and baseball.

We stopped for a lunch break on a wide place in the trail, where a rising cliff was at our backs, and a sharp long drop to the river in front of us. Bill was making notes in the margins of his maps, and taking photographs. I decided this was as good a time as any to brace him.

"Bill, I am more than content to be making this trek with you, and I surely do enjoy your company, but it's time for you to level with me. This business of field-testing your pack is hogwash. What kind of intelligence-gathering mission are you on?"

Bill looked briefly away, then turned and met my eyes.

"Steve, of course nobody expects you to believe that cover story. And of course it's pretty obvious. Your realize that, with the situation in Asia as it now is, Nepal could become an extremely strategic area at any time, especially given the large number of Chinese troops who are held down in the occupation of Tibet. The small, but continuing, Tibetan guerilla resistance to the Chinese, and the presence of the Dalai Lama in India, and the Tibetan refugee camps in both Nepal and India, make things even more complex and unstable. While 'certain Agencies of the U.S. government' are providing training and minor tangible support to the Tibetan resistance, we know very little about the detailed geography of Nepal from the ground level. My assignment is to scope out this particular route in case we should ever have need to use it, and to learn a little about the country for general purposes. Obviously, Nepal might become important to our national interests vis-a-vis China in the event of possible contingencies. I have appreciated your discretion about this as we've traveled along together, and that's all I can tell you."

He would say no more, and the discussion turned to the personal generalities of our individual lives.

That last evening before reaching Pokhara, we came upon a *Thakali bhatti* along the trail. The Thakalis are a tribe of the northern hills, restless wanderers but natural traders and merchants. They have been important intermediaries in the salt-for-wool trade that has linked India and Tibet since time immemorial. Along the main trade routes, Thakali women would set up *bhattis* (literally, "rice places") where the best tea, rice, fruits in season, cigarettes and biscuits from India, and even fresh eggs, were to be had. Porters and trail travelers would gather there, for the food, the *rakshi*, the gambling, and perhaps for other less-mentionable forms of entertainment. We had a marvelous meal of rice and eggs, swigged down the tea, and spread our bags just beyond the edge of the firelight. The singing and laughter of the porters eased us to sleep; the night was cool and dry, the stars were down close upon us, and there is no sleep better in the world than that.

We were close to Pokhara now, entering the soft green valley on that last morning. As we moved up the valley, we had to ford a stream, full and swift moving from the recent monsoon, but not overflowing. We were smooth and easy with the rhythm of four days on the trail, and our packs felt like weightless extensions of ourselves.

The sun was warm and gentle on our right shoulders as we waded into the stream, alongside each other and about 10 yards apart.

I heard the dry "pop" that sounds like exactly what it is, followed by Bill's cry of pain, and saw him drop to one knee in the stream. "Goddamn it to hell, I've rolled my foot over on a loose stone, and busted my ankle," he diagnosed even before I reached him.

I helped him hop out of the far side of the stream, pulled up his left pant-leg, took off his boot and sock (THAT was not much fun for him, I tell you), and examined the rapidly swelling and discoloring area on the outside of his left ankle. That done, I put his left leg back in the cold water of the stream, to try and get what little help we could to reduce the rate of swelling.

"What's the deal, Doc? It rightly smarts."

"Okay, Bill. You have indeed, at the least, knocked a chip out of what we call your lateral malleolus. Also obviously torn, or badly strained, some ligaments. I don't think you have a major fracture, Major, but an x-ray will be needed to tell us that, and you sure are not going on any jaunt up north to Jomosom any time soon. We are just lucky we are only about three miles short of the Pokhara airstrip, and there is a daily flight to Kathmandu. We can sit and drink almost-real whiskey at what passes for the airport hotel while we wait for the plane. Probably, no ice available, though, neither for your ankle nor for the whiskey."

"That's not good enough, Doc. Let me just sit here and think for a minute, and then we need to talk."

"Okay, but let me give you some painkiller by mouth, and strap up your ankle, before we do anything else."

"Nope, I need as clear a head as I can get. We have a problem. Get started wrapping the ankle, but hold the jolly pills until I figure things out." He was reverting to his usual field command personality.

I was not following his line of thought completely, but if that's what he wanted . . .

I dug out an ACE bandage and some adhesive tape. I cut off the end of his pant-leg, cut some short slits in the top of his left boot, one on each side. I then hunted up a thin stick, flat as I could find, and also cut a long stout stick that he could use to hobble on. We had several miles to go over uneven ground, and I knew the ankle would continue to swell. I did not want to constrict it too much. At the back of my mind was a concern that the ankle might be more badly broken than I thought, which is always a danger with ankle injuries, and that it would be good to get him back to Kathmandu quickly, on the afternoon plane if possible. My other alternative was to go for help, round up a couple of porters, and even perhaps have him carried up to the Shining Hospital, a British missionary outfit about a dozen miles away, beyond the north end of Pokhara. It seemed to me a crap-shoot, but that my chosen course was the better one. I was conscious that this was a pretty tough bird who could probably handle a few miles of pain at the hobble, and I wanted him to have the best care possible, given his chosen profession.

I wrapped and strapped his ankle, but not too tightly, broke the flat stick in two and taped it on firmly on each side of the ankle as a splint, slid on his slit boot, and sat back to hear what he had to say.

Bill took a sip from his canteen, looked me in the eye, and let fly without blinking. "Steve, I really haven't leveled with you, wasn't supposed to, and now I guess I have to. I really appreciate your coming with me this far. What you weren't supposed to know is that there was, or is, a second part to the mission, one that is confidential and that I was going to do solo up north, leaving you to fly home from here in Pokhara.

"Sometime in the next few days, the Khambas are bringing down an important person from Tibet, sneaking him past the Chinese out over a small pass west of Mustang, and down a back trail behind Marpha and Jomosom, over by the Dhaulagiri massif."

So, it seemed that Mister Major Thompson indeed knew a lot more about the geography of Nepal than had been apparent.

Bill continued, "He is apparently an incarnation of some important Lama. My assignment is to link up with the Tibetans here on the Nepalese side, show the flag for the U.S. and perhaps accompany him on to the main Tibetan refuge-in-exile in India. Given what is going on in Asia, we view it as very important to begin to develop strong positive relationships with the Khambas, and with the Tibetans in general. There is a very narrow window of timing for the mission; the Chinese will certainly be after him as soon as he is missed in Lhasa, and they will most probably try to intercept him at the frontier, or even maybe cross into Nepalese territory ahead of him. I need to complete my mission."

I replied, "Well, if you can grow wings in the next twenty-four hours, or swim up the creeks and rivers, I guess you might be able to. But otherwise, no way. No way. This isn't about your willpower or your self-discipline. You just don't have the physical equipment, and won't have for a month. Sorry, but that's the way it is."

He thought for a moment. "Okay, Doc. Then you have to do it."

My jaw dropped, and I thought of the good and sufficient reasons why I couldn't and shouldn't. I really didn't know what was going on here. To take an active role in what clearly appeared to be a military and intelligence operation could get me, and the Peace Corps, in a world of trouble. Then I thought a little more, about myself, and about what other Americans were doing that they couldn't or shouldn't do, in other places in the world. How could, or should, I do less? Where was the greater obligation? Was not, as Hippocrates said, "experience treacherous and judgement difficult?" How could I know which decision was the right one to take?

Then I said, "Okay, if that's what's needed, let's get on with it. First stop Pokhara airstrip."

I gave Bill a couple of Darvons, plenty of water, and we hobbled our way to Pokhara. Neither of us said much along the way.

We had a couple of hours before the afternoon plane from Kathmandu was due to come in and turn around, so we sat back in the outdoor "restaurant" of the grass-strip airport bungalow hotel and coughed up a lot of rupees for a bottle of Indian "Scotch." Bill had gotten a seat on the plane, and I asked the dispatcher to have the pilot radio ahead to have an Embassy car meet Bill when they landed in Kathmandu. After the hop up from the stream to the airstrip, the ankle was quite swollen, and must have hurt more than a little, but Bill was in pretty good shape. The whiskey was probably doing him more good than the Darvon was, though the combination of the two can sometimes be wicked. Florence, the Embassy nurse, would know how to get him to Shanta Bhawan Mission Hospital in Kathmandu, and I expected he would be all right from that point on.

There wasn't much else to brief me on. He was expected, the next day or the day after at the latest, not at all the same thing as *bohli-parsi*, at the Tibetan refugee camp less than 10 miles west of Pokhara. There someone would make himself known to him, using the password, "It is a long way to India," and Bill was to reply, "But shorter than to Beijing." From that point on he would be given further instructions concerning the route and the meeting with the escaping Tibetans further north. "They'll be expecting ME, of course, but you should be all right as long as you have the passwords. We gringos probably all look the same to the Tibetans, anyway."

Then Bill, after looking around and ascertaining that we were alone in the patio, said, "There's one more thing I didn't tell you about either, Steve. I really don't know what might come up on the trail, or what might go down with the Chinese. You better take this." He passed me a cloth-wrapped small bundle from his pack. I peeked inside, and there was the Army's favorite Colt APC 45 caliber automatic pistol in an Army-issue holster with an extra ammo clip in a small pouch on the holster front. I just looked at him. This was getting crazier by the minute. I could think of nothing to say, so I just shook my head and slid the pistol into my pack.

Bill said, "Better to have it, and not be without it if you should want it. Know how to use it?" I nodded my head once, which in the U.S. means "yes," but in Nepal means "no," and remained silent.

"The Chinese will be serious about this. They will have armed patrols, either in Tibet or, perhaps, illegally within Nepalese territory, and they won't be asking to see anybody's passports. Hopefully, both you and the Tibetan Lama's party will be able to evade them, but if you come across them, they will either take you prisoner or shoot you, and there won't be any witnesses or anyone to help you up on the frontier. The Nepalis won't want to know anything about it, even if, as is possible, they have looked the other way and informally allowed the Chinese searchers to come over the border. For little Nepal, it's best not to see and not to know—not to get involved."

In for a penny, in for a pound? That seemed easy to say, but harder to come to terms with. But I was in it now, and could see no other course for myself but to go forward.

Bill's plane was pretty much on time. I helped him across the runway, up the movable stairs, and into his seat. We still didn't say much. I knew he was thinking about the mission, and about his upcoming next assignment, which he had told me was to be in Special Ops in Vietnam. I hoped he would heal fast enough and well enough to keep it, because he wanted it. We shook hands and said goodbye. I turned my head away as the propellers kicked up dust from the dirt-strip runway. I never saw that Kentucky boy again.

We had six PCVs, in three households, in Pokhara town, and I spent the rest of the day and that evening with them. I was pretty beat when I got to sleep in one of the PCV houses, and I can't remember what story I gave them about the reason for my trip further north and west. At that time, the farthest north and west of Pokhara that we had volunteers stationed was at Baglung, and I would be passing through Baglung, so I must have concocted something credible around that.

Pokhara bazaar is stretched out and seems to go on forever; it was almost mid-morning by the time I got clear of the last houses and passed by the Shining Hospital. I didn't stop; I saw no use leaving more traces than I had to. I just kept on along the shore of Lake Piuwital. There was a festival in progress. There is always a festival in progress in Nepal, most every day of the year. A group of young Nepali girls wrapped in shimmering pastel dresses with flowing skirts and billowing long sleeves, was dancing on the lakeshore. They looked like beautiful, graceful butterflies skimming on the breeze. I thought of Bill's mission, my mission lying ahead of me, and shook my head and swallowed hard at the contrast.

About noon I came to the sprawling Tibetan refugee camp. Without anything better in mind, I made my way to the health post run by a young Italian doctor I knew slightly. "How good to see you," he said, and a young Tibetan woman rolling bandages added, "Yes, it is a long way to India."

I wasn't sure whether to look at her or at him, and I replied, "But shorter than to Beijing." They both smiled.

The doctor said, "We were expecting someone else, a Major

Thompson. Aren't you the Peace Corps doctor?" I explained the switch to him, which was probably a bit easier than it might have been, since he was a physician and I was not a stranger to him. He smiled again, and said, "Let me take you to Dolma."

Dolma was friendly, but obviously a hard case, with the black wool Tibetan robe, high boots, and short sword stuck through his red sash. His long black hair was braided and coiled on top of his head, adding to his six feet of height. His scraggly sparse black beard and long mustache set off mahogany cheekbones and obsidian eyes.

He listened to the story, shook his head, and said, in excellent English, "Well, we'll just have to do what we can with what we have. Here's the plan. We know from our own spies that the Chinese have covered the major passes, and sent patrols on the trails inside Nepalese territory as a fail-safe. We'll take care of the latter as we find them, but we can't engage the frontier troops."

"How will it be possible to avoid being spotted by the Chinese?" I asked Dolma.

"Our gamble is that the seldom-used Pindu La (pass) won't be covered, as are the major passes around Mustang, and that by taking the longer trails around the back side of Dhauligiri our party can sneak through. Certainly the Nepalese Army won't be up there. Once the group gets below Jomosom they should be relatively safe, unless the Nepalese turn them back. If you insist on meeting them above or near Jomosom, you go ahead now, and I will follow late tomorrow or early the next day, in case any further message comes in here by runner that would change the situation."

He recited both to himself and to me, as if he were reading from a lesson plan, as his finger traced a route on the map. "Let's see, it will take you about three or three and a half days to reach a point above Marpha by this indirect route: northwest, up the Mayandi Khola, then north into the Himal behind Dhauligiri, and then swinging back east to come at the west bank of the Kali Ghandaki Khola at Marpha, and up past Jomosom, which will be hidden from you, and you from it, on the opposite east bank. But under no circumstances should you go through Jomosom, or even up the main Kali Ghandaki trail on the Jomosom side of the river. Stay on the Marpha side. That's the reason you are going up the long way around Dhaulagiri. Jomosom has a police post, and we can't risk getting intercepted up so close to the Tibetan border; the Nepalis might send us back into the hands of the Chinese."

He stabbed his finger onto a point on the map. "I will meet up with you along the trail somewhere about here, late in the afternoon four days from now, or the next morning after that. If you meet up with them before I get to you, you will certainly recognize them, and they won't have any trouble recognizing you. Or you can wait here in Pokhara, and we'll bring them down to you."

"The mission is to link up above Marpha, those are my instructions. I'd better go ahead," I replied.

"Travel well, then. The passwords are the same. I will see you up north."

5

It was a lovely walk along the valley from Pokhara towards Baglung, especially now, in the early autumn just after the monsoons. The paddies were green with ripening stalks of rice. There were tall cones of haystacks set high on posts and platforms to keep the rats off. The reddish mud-and-wattle thatched-roof houses of the small villages were decorated with whitewash accents and designs. The incredibly high and impossibly white snow masses of the Annapurna range loomed over me, with a sky so blue behind them that it made my heart ache. Toward the north, standing seemingly apart, rose the sharp 22,000 foot snow peak of Machupuchhare, whose unmistakable and unforgettable split "fish tail" summit came into view as I moved around to a perspective of its southwestern side. Children and dogs ran out of the villages, following me up the trail as I passed. The children pointed and laughed and shouted and sang, some of them trying out their best school English.

"Sir, Mister, where going you to? Give *paisa*. Where you are from? Take me to America!"

Several hours from the Tibetan camp, about as long as it took me to eat a half-kilo of ripe *suntalas* purchased at the trailside, I came to the major trail junction at Naudanda, where the main trail heads due north up the east side of the mighty Kali Ghandaki river. Some say that the gorge of the Kali Ghandaki is the deepest gorge in the world, because the river passes between the two gigantic highest peaks of the Annapurna and Dhauligiri massifs, each over 24,000 feet high. The river and its gorge separate the two peaks, which are less than 20 miles apart at their summits, and the drop from the summits to the river is about 18 thousand feet. This is a vertical distance of almost three and a half miles, or about three times the depth of the Grand Canyon of the Colorado.

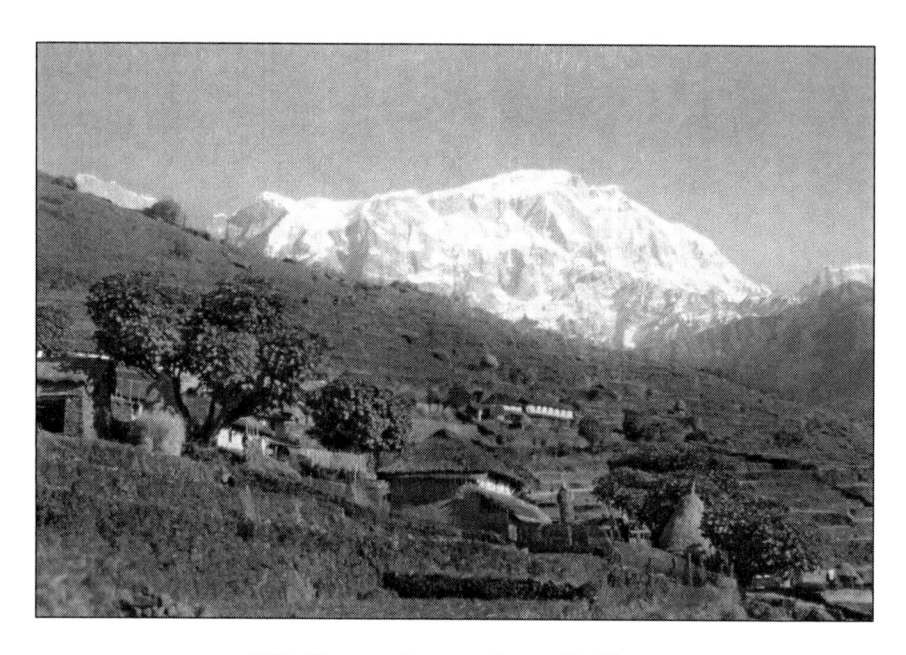

Hill villages and terraces beyond Pokhara

The goddess Kali, for whom the river and the gorge are named, is, among other things, the keeper and eater of dead souls, and the Black Kali is the evocation of smallpox. But I was not heading up the Kali Ghandaki, though I had been in that amazing gorge on previous occasions. Some sections of the trail are blasted out from the face of the sheer cliff, hanging above the mighty river. After climbing up the ridge near Naudanda, I was heading on west to the village of Baglung, the second ridge, upon which it sat, now just appearing in the distance. The east bank of the Kali Ghandaki, the main trail to Jomosom, would have been a much easier and shorter way to go, but since the Tibetan party was coming down the "back way." I could not take a chance of our missing each other, and so had to head up the circuitous route to intersect them if we should meet either up- or down-stream from Marpha. Besides, it was wise for us to bypass Jomosom, which would undoubtedly have a police, if not a Nepali Army, post along the trail. Marpha, which is on the west side of the Kali, is screened from Jomosom, which lies on the east side of the river, by a steep ridge. The Tibetans, who were supposedly coming down via the little-used Pindu La pass, could come directly via a secondary trail through Marpha, on the west side of the river, and have a better chance of never being spotted or intercepted from Jomosom.

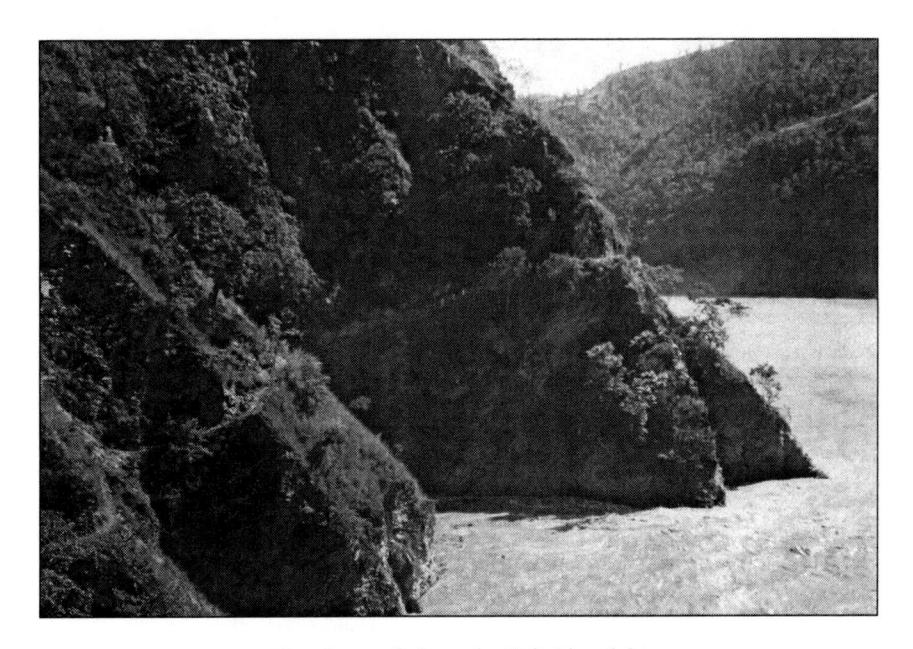

Hanging trail along the Kali Ghandaki

We had two volunteers living in Baglung, and I stopped the night with them. One had a nasty and painful boil on the inner part of his right thigh. By the light of a kerosene lantern I lanced it, stuck a wick of iodoform gauze in as a drain, smeared on some antibiotic ointment, and put on a small dressing. I told him to pull the wick in four days, or to go to Shining Hospital if the wound became infected, which I was sure it would not.

The other PCV seemed in good shape, but he took me aside.

"Doc, I'm feeling pretty good about things, love living and teaching English here. But you know Maggie, the volunteer down in Pokhara? We get together whenever we can, and, you know, we're sort of fooling around."

I gave him a stack of condoms and said, "Be careful, and think about what you're doing."

"You won't tell Willi or anybody in the office, will you?" he asked.

"Oh, yes, of course I will. I'll tell each and every one, and I'll write a letter to your Mama, too," I reassured him.

At that time, Baglung and the small Gurung village of Siklis a few hours walk beyond it were the furthest points west and north from Kathmandu where we had volunteers stationed. Anything further out was considered to be too remote for safety. In the morning, I told the PCVs that I was going to swing through Siklis and then directly back down to Pokhara. I knew that Ray, the lone volunteer in Siklis, was away on leave in Thailand, and thus the fact that I had never, in fact, visited him that day would not get back to Baglung or to Pokhara.

I walked through the village of Beni, and now was in territory that I had never before passed through. I headed northwest as if towards far Dhorpatan and on to Dolpo, but I was actually planning to turn off near Dharapani and then bear north to thread the needle between the peaks of the Dhaulagiri range. I knew that I had a couple of difficult days on the trail ahead of me, but I was feeling confident, and in good trail shape. Bill had given me some extra dry rations and a small spirit stove he had secreted in his pack, and I had borrowed a thick sweater from the Italian doctor, as well as a pound of rice. There would be plenty of water for rice and tea, and the sky looked as if the weather would hold fair. Nevertheless, I would have to climb up above 15,000 feet to cross the Thapa La pass, and there was always the chance of bad weather, or an early-season snowstorm messing up my plans, and possibly getting me into real trouble.

Around mid-day, having made good time and passed beyond Dharapani, I found that I needed to ford two good-sized watercourses, feeders to the Mayandi Khola, itself a tributary of the mighty Kali.

The first stream did not pose a major problem, and I crossed without incident. But the second, more a small river than a stream, was another matter.

It was perhaps forty feet wide, and tumbling swiftly. The water was opaque and milky gray from glacial silt and debris carried down from the high mountains beyond. The water was icy, and as I stood on the bank I could hear the grumbling and grinding of stones as they milled against each other in the current. I had no walking staff with me, and was now above the terrain where it would be easy to find or cut one large enough to be of use.

As if to add a warning, clouds suddenly blew in on a chill wind, and obscured the sun. I had no way to reliably estimate the river's depth, nor to look for a shallow place to cross, one without deep and unexpected holes.

A phrase from my old Wyoming trail boss, Billy Jiggs, came to mind: *What you gotta do, you just gotta do it. Cowboy up, Mister.*

I knew it was courting disaster to try and cross with my heavy pack on. I took it off, opened it, and wrapped the water-sensitive contents snugly in the ground cloth which I then tied in a tight bundle with a short section of parachute cord. I closed the lashings of the pack as tight as I could get them, and then tied one end of the remaining ninety feet of parachute cord securely to the pack's external frame. I left the sleeping bag in its lashings on the outside of the pack, reasoning that the down-filled bag would increase flotation, and that the contents of the pack, and the air spaces within it, would quite likely add up to a total bundle that would not sink, at least until things became heavily waterlogged. I had taken from the pack only my matches in their waterproof safe, and my compass, and stored them securely in my buttoned pockets. If worst came to worst, I could survive and find my way to safety with only those items and a knife, I assumed. All the rest stayed in the pack, except for my Swiss Army Knife, which I slid, long blade opened, inside my shirt.

After cutting off 10 feet or so from the parachute cord for another use, I tied the free end of the cord as securely as I could around the corners of a rough stone of about three pounds' weight, pulling the knots tight after soaking them in the water. Then I heaved the rock, with the cord attached, across the river, with a grenade-style motion. It landed on the far bank with a satisfying clunk, and the light loose cord bellied out before it, floating on the surface of the water, without great tension between the stone on the far bank and the pack at my feet. There seemed no danger that the current would pull either the stone or the pack into the water.

I tied each of my bootlaces in a single tight bow. Using four other very short pieces of parachute cord from the length I had previously cut, I tied off my pants' and shirt's cuffs, so that whatever little air was trapped inside would add to my buoyancy. I gave myself only a slight chance of cutting free of my boots with the Swiss Army knife if I was swept away, but I figured every little bit I could do for myself would be of help. There was surely no one else who was going to help me. The alternative would have been to remove boots and socks, and hang them around my neck, but the temperature of the water, and, more importantly, the rolling, growling rocks in the riverbed made going barefoot impracticable and even more unsafe for a crossing.

I moved about fifty yards upstream from the floating parachute cord, thinking that if I did get swept away I might grab onto it as I went by, and use the pack as an anchor.

Here we go, Buster. Last one in is a rotten egg. I stepped cautiously into the river, feeling with my boots for loose rocks that might roll me off balance.

At first, all went well, and I suppose I got a little cocky and tried to move too fast. The invisible riverbed began to deepen rapidly, increasing the pressure of the current against my thighs, and I could feel the stones moving beneath my boots, giving no solid purchase.

The next thing that I knew, I was in the water, my head submerged with the rest of me, tossing and tumbling in the current, banging on rocks as I went by. By instinct, I shielded my head with my arms to protect it, and somehow simultaneously curled my body and kicked as strongly as I could, in which direction, I was entirely unaware.

There is that old story about "your whole life passing slowly before your eyes" when you are drowning or falling from a great height. That's not the way it was for me. For me, it was as if there were two separate rolls of motion picture film running at the same time, each of which I could observe and comprehend. The first was an inchoate, breathless, terrifying bashing of my body hurtling down the river. There was no up, no down, it was as if everything was rushing *by me*, rather than vice versa. But at the same time I was acutely conscious of myself straining, slowly, slowly, and as if against a great weight, to push across the current and against the river, if indeed I could guess which was the direction in which to push. There was terror, and there was effort. Nothing else. No pain, no thought of past or future. All was in the present.

I found myself lying on the far bank, gasping and retching, my body stretched on the stony ground and my boots still being lapped by the water. I had absolutely no understanding of how I had gotten there. Apart from a few bruises, none on my head, I seemed unhurt. When I was able to lift myself to my knees and look around, I saw in the distance the cord, still floating in a convex bend aimed at me, in the current, and the pack still lying secure on the opposite shore. I judged that I had traveled perhaps two hundred yards downstream, and that everything else within sight, except for the moving current, was, and had been, soundless and still. It was as if I had stepped out of a room, and then stepped back in again through a different door.

It came to me suddenly how cold I was, and I began to shiver. It was a few moments work to draw the pack across the river with the parachute cord, and the pack did indeed float.

Beating my arms against my body, and dancing up and down, I gathered enough twigs and dry small monsoon driftwood from the riverbank and beyond. I made fire, a very small one, stripped off my clothes, covered myself with the mostly dry ground cloth from within the pack, and curled, like an exhausted and hunted animal, close around the fire.

As I warmed, and conscious thought returned, fear came with it. I began to shake violently again, this time not from cold, but from the terror of what might have been. I heard myself singing, wordless crooning from a time before speech existed. I may have prayed, but, if so, it would have been to the spirits of the river and of the rocks.

Later, I don't know how much later, I was warm, relatively dry in odd pieces of spare clothing, hungry to eat some dry rations from the pack, and drink water from a re-filled canteen. I grinned wolfishly at the spectacle of drinking the water that had so recently tried to drown me, and I thought of an old saying: *When you meet the bear, either you eat the bear, or the bear eats you.* I built the fire up higher, spread out my wet clothing and the sodden sleeping bag to dry before it, and lay back against the pack.

The pack? Suddenly I realized the mistake I had made. Dummy! What I should have done was to take the time to test the pack for flotation at the edge of the river, and tied myself to it with the long cord as a safety line, with the knife handy for emergency escape. Then I could have grabbed hold of the pack like a kickboard, and kicked my way diagonally across the current, safe from the hazards on the riverbed. I might have gone a fair way further downstream, but I would have been much safer doing it. Failing that, if I was determined to cross on foot, I should have gone back a half-mile, or whatever, to where I could have cut a staff. Why was I always in such a goddamn hurry!

Of course, the pack might not have adequately buoyed my weight, or might have taken in water and sunk, and I would have drowned. It is often difficult, even after the fact, to know which road is the better one to choose.

It was now well into the afternoon, and I decided to stay the night where I was at the riverside. My things needed some more drying out, and I was sore and shaken. I didn't know the country ahead, but the map showed few, if any, villages of any size. I would be headed toward the most difficult part of the journey, the high and cold country, mostly uninhabited, between the peaks of the Dhaulagiri range. I needed to be in the best shape possible for that. I could make up the time I had lost by staying put now, I reasoned, by traveling at night beyond Marpha as I came eastward out of the high country, and then turned north along the west bank of the Kali. I took some aspirin for my soreness and stiffness, built the fire up high, boiled up some rice and some strong tea, and put on my sweater and a pair of dry socks. I rolled myself in the groundsheet next to the fire, which now was banked for the night, and was soon asleep.

In dreams that night I was floating in the current, slowly and aimlessly, down a warm river. There was no discomfort, no obvious danger. But I knew that I would float alone on that river, forever and forever, down through darkness with no borders and no ending. And no one would ever know where I was, or where I had been.

I awoke from the dream, and the stars were crystal clear and unforgivingly cold above me, far away, remote, impersonal and uncaring. They were not at all the same stars of the nights on the trail with Bill between Tansen and Pokhara.

The decision to lose time now, and then to make it up by traveling at night later on beyond Marpha, probably saved my life in the encounter that was to come.

The day broke with clear sunshine, sparkling like diamonds from the snow peaks that lay before me in a semi-circle to the north. From where I stood it was impossible to pick out the narrow valley that would lead me between Dhaulagiri One and the only slightly lower secondary peaks to its west. I had some cold rice, biscuits, and river water, humped my load, and moved off. My feelings were of mixed anticipation and trepidation. Would I be able to climb the high valley and surmount the pass? Would the fine weather hold? Would I meet the Tibetans as planned, and perhaps even meet them well on "my side," the south side, of the pass, thus avoiding the hardest challenge?

I kept thinking of Bill Thompson, rolling his ankle on a little stone, and what that would mean if the same happened to me up here. I was afraid, but I was exhilarated by these Shining Mountains, these Himalayas, awaiting me. I felt strangely rested and fit, with little residual stiffness from my river ordeal of yesterday.

In the event, the day's dangers never materialized, and I passed the hours in a fantasy world that still takes my breath away when I think about it. The trail rose steadily over rocky mountainous terrain, but somewhat gradually. There were abandoned stone huts in short blue-green grass pastures. At the few small villages I passed there were yaks, and the people, who were themselves few in number, stared at me as if I came from another world, which indeed I did. They spoke a language of which I comprehended only one word, and they, equally, could not understand my speech. But they smiled, and offered me hot tea with yak butter, and I smiled, and gave them Indian sweets and machine-rolled cigarettes. They always pointed up the valley, and repeated that one word: "*La. La. La.*" The Pass, as if to tell me that all depended on that. They stood, watching me, until we faded from one another through the distance.

The mountain walls rose, and rose, and rose again, on either side of me. The sky became narrow between them. I felt that I was again in a river, but this time carried along by one that nurtured and protected me, that gathered me up in its arms, and made for me a pathway to heaven.

For periods I walked with my arms spread up and out wide, singing and shouting, and hearing the echoes respond. I remembered the old words, "... though I walk through the Valley of the Shadow of Death, I shall fear no Evil...." On this day, there was no Evil here.

I slept that night at the foot of the Thapa La, in a ruined stone roofless hut, near to a prayer wall, a *Mani* wall. Amongst the stones were some that had been chiseled, with infinite patient delicacy, in a strange script blackened over with charcoal. I knew what it said: "*Om mani padme hum.*" The jewel is in the lotus. The snow mountains shone with their own light. The strip of sky was so narrow that I could make out no constellations. There was no moon.

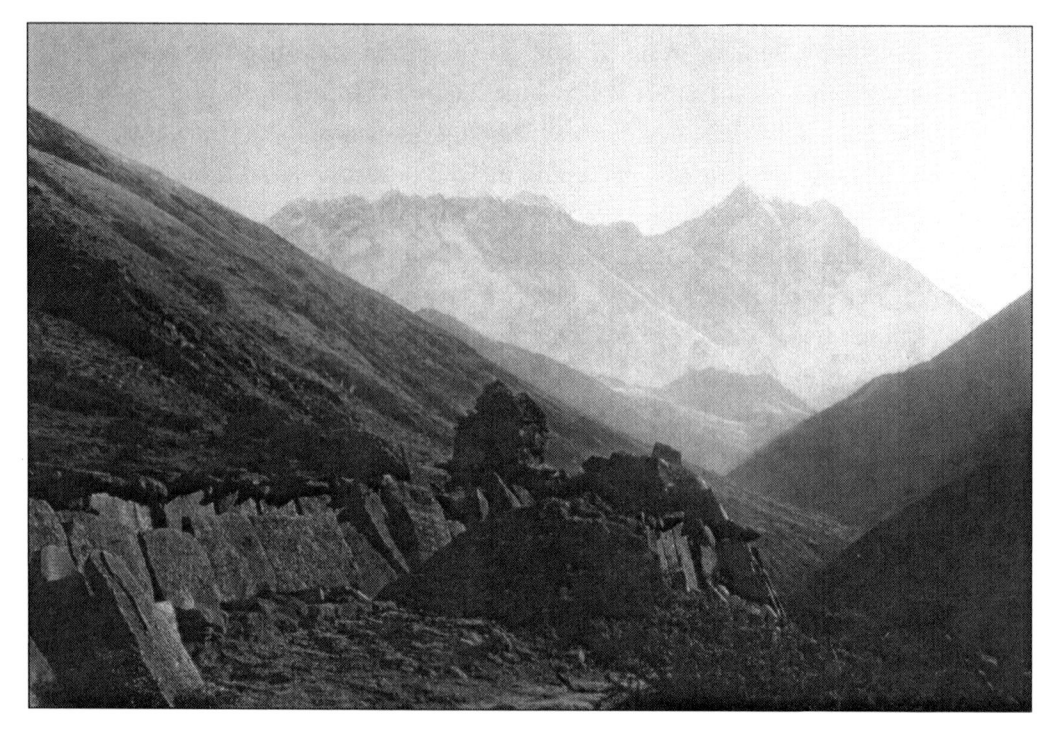

Mani wall near the pass

I awoke to a frozen tiny stream in the valley, and fresh frost that indicated light snow higher up. I felt no sense of danger, only of wonder, as I threw on my pack, which seemed weightless even at this altitude, and started up. Not having packed for high altitude snow country, I had only two shirts and a sweater, no gloves, and a baseball cap that said "Jackson Hole, Wyoming" in red letters.

I felt no cold. I felt no fear. I felt no longing but for the intimate solitude of this day, and this place.

It was slow going in the thin air as I mounted the Thapa La. As I rose higher and higher, the world spread out before me. Peaks and peaks and still more peaks, now all around me, an ocean of peaks as far as I could see. As I came to the top of the pass, there was snow on the ground. *Mani* walls guarded the approaches. Prayer flags, faded and tattered by the winds of uncounted seasons, rapped and snapped in the stiff breeze. On the very crest of the La was a cairn of loose stones, higher than a man and broader than a yak. As had each passer-by for a thousand years, I bent, picked up a stone, and added it to the cairn. I rested for a while, lost in thought, but the wind cut sharply, and soon I turned my feet to the east, and descended the pass, toward Marpha.

I came down upon Marpha, beyond which I could see the rolling of the mighty Kali Ghandaki, in mid-afternoon. I decided that it would be best to wait several hours, and then to walk through Marpha after dark. Then, if there was no sign of the Tibetan party, I would continue upstream along the west bank of the river, swinging westward along the trail that they should be coming down towards me.

Upstream of Marpha and Jomosom, I would pass through a great gate in the mountains. The Annnapurna and Dhaulagiri ranges would now be to the south, and I would find myself on a high, desert-like plateau, swept by the strong winds that then funnel into the Kali Ghandaki gorge. In all respects save political boundaries, I would be at the southern pillars that hold up the roof of the world, though there would still be much elevation to gain, foot by foot, to reach the passes through the great mountains and to stand in Tibet.

The houses now were flat-roofed, made of stone. Prayer flags flew everywhere. The people were tall and lean, and many more spoke Tibetan than Nepali. Their dress was the robes and aprons and tall boots of the Tibetan plateau. No rice was grown, just the tall grains of colder climates. There were many Thakalis living here, but more people who had been displaced, either recently or a hundred years ago, from further north, in Tibet.

I stopped at a tea house on the outskirts of Marpha, and found someone who could speak Nepali with me. His Nepali may have been as broken and ungrammatical as my own.

"*Bhoti manche anu hos aju ya hijo, Dadju?*" (Have Tibetans come by here today or yesterday, Elder Brother?)

"*Dherai Bhoti bata janu, tara pani aju, Bhai!*" (Many Tibetans pass by here, but none today, Younger Brother.)

So they were still above me, to the north and west, headed toward me, unless they had been taken by the Chinese, or had come to grief on the high pass, or one of a thousand other possible misfortunes had befallen them on their journey.

I decided to follow my plan, and to move along in the dark. After I left Marpha, realizing that it was unlikely that I would meet innocent stray travelers on the trail, I resolved to go very carefully and as quietly as I could. Within several hours, I approached the trail junction that led, to the east, across the Kali Ghandaki to Muktinath. To the north, it aimed up towards Mustang and the main pass, the Syawala La, into Tibet. To the west, the direction that I would now take, it headed off toward the more remote and less-used Pindu La pass that the party I was seeking to intercept was planning to traverse.

Moving ahead slowly in semi-darkness lit only by the stars, I heard, against the background of silence, the sound of a man pissing on a flat rock.

The sound was unmistakable. I stopped dead still in my tracks, and strained my eyes toward what I was hearing. Dimly, in the starlight, I could make out a figure, his back to me, concentrating, chin down, on passing urine. I was sure that he was in uniform, and that his short-peaked cap was Chinese, and certainly not of the Nepali army or police. Looking more closely, I could see at his right side, propped against a boulder, the green glow of what I took to be a military short-wave radio set. Next to it stood the skeleton-like silhouette of a rifle.

What if he had been facing me, instead of turned away? What if he had been looking up, instead of down? What if he had already been doing up his buttons, and had been surrounded closely by the silence of the night? What if I had been mistaken, and he was Nepalese? What if he had not been, as he seemed to be, a lone outposted scout, and if there had been other soldiers in the rocks around him? What if we had come upon each other by daylight?

As silently and slowly as I could, I backed step by step down the way I had come. At a distance of a hundred paces, counted off by half the thundering beating of my heart, I stopped, and silently took off my pack. Opening one corner of the top flap, I drew the cloth-wrapped automatic pistol. Feeling with my fingers that the clip was in place, I curled my body around the Colt, muffling the sound of racking a round into the chamber. Taking off the safety made no sound at all.

Standing absolutely still, I took stock of my situation. If I stayed here, or backed further away, he would discover me, or intercept the Tibetans as they came down, in daylight. If I backed off, in effect turning and running away, abandoning the mission, I would leave the Tibetans to the mercy of capture by the Chinese. I couldn't do that. If I tried to sneak around him by going off the trail in the darkness, and he discovered me, I would be badly outgunned: my pistol against his automatic rifle. If I rushed him, the noise would alert him, and again, I would be badly out-matched. If, somehow, I could overpower him, what would I do with him? I wasn't in a position to take or keep him prisoner, and if, in any of these instances, he was able to use his radio, the game was up entirely. Convinced that if I moved off the trail into the loose rocks on either side I would alert the Chinese soldier, I very slowly inched my way back up towards him on the trail, guiding myself by the glow of his cigarette.

I moved, stopped, moved again, stopped again, and came within 20 feet of him. His body was turned half-sideways to me. Only later did I ask myself what I had decided to do. Was I planning to take him prisoner, tie him up, and turn off his radio? Unlikely that this would have worked, and what, in the end, would I have done with him?

I think now that when I drew that pistol, I must have made the decision to use it.

Some sound, or perhaps a sixth sense, alerted him. He gave an exclamation, spat out his cigarette, and turned and started toward me, his right arm grasping for the rifle.

I shot him, once and then once again, and saw the impact against his chest. He gave a soft grunt, and then a long hiss of air. Turning half away from me, he raised his left arm, as if in supplication or defense, and I shot him again. "Ahhhh," he said, and bending at the waist, sunk to his knees and curled to the ground.

I was numbed, but also conscious of every detail, as if I was once again tumbling in the river. He was so still that I knew he was dead, and when I came close to him, his eyes were fully open and unmoving. I made sure that there was no breathing, no pulse, and no reaction of his wide pupils before I put the safety back on the pistol. Then I went back down the trail to retrieve my pack.

Going over him with my small flashlight, I saw that he was not much more than a child, perhaps sixteen, but perhaps I misjudged his age. One bullet had torn through the breast of his uniform, a small hole no bigger than one of his uniform buttons, and had exited his back with a hole the size of your fist. The second shot must have gone wide, and traveled wherever missed shots go. My third shot, when he had raised his arm, had gone in just below his left armpit. My clinical eye, operating on automatic pilot, guessed that the bullet had ripped open a major vessel in the chest, probably one of the Great Vessels clustered at the base of the heart. His mouth was half-open, and pouring from it onto the ground before him, and spilled over his uniform tunic, was more blood than you can imagine. In the glow of the flashlight, the blood was as black as the heart of Kali herself. No tint of red, just black.

I turned off the field radio, and left it where it was. I picked up the short assault rifle that had fallen from his hand, and put it down again, flat behind a large rock. The body of the Young Chinese Soldier (for that is what I came to call him, in the dreams and waking hours of my future life), I rolled off the other side of the trail, where there was a steep drop, and I pitched the radio over after it. I scuffed the rocky ground as best I could to cover the blood sign, but I knew that by dawn the gathering of ravens would mark the spot.

Thinking/Not thinking, I moved forward up the trail a quarter mile, so that anyone coming down to look for the Young Chinese Soldier would blunder into me before finding any sign of him.

Then I put down the cocked pistol before me on a large rock, safety on, and sat down to wait for whatever daylight would bring. I did not sleep, not that I was aware of. At least one small dark corner of my soul now belonged to Kali, and perhaps always had.

I am a doctor, not a killer. But now I am a killer who is also a doctor.

Dawn came, the sun rose, the birds sang. Ravens circled behind and below me, rasping their magic calls. I sipped water from the canteen, but felt no hunger.

After a while, I heard the tinkling of bells coming up the trail from behind me. From far off I heard it, and then it came closer, toward me. It stopped for a bit, and then came closer still.

Dolma was leading a single horse, packed lightly. The small, shaggy pony was the Tibetan kind, the kind that can go anywhere, at any altitude, and just keep going. In the north of Nepal you would hear those pony trains, led by traders or smugglers, or both, coming from far away, and hear the jingle of those bells long before you heard the creak of the harness. On they would come, then pass you, and the bells would fade slowly into the distance.

I pushed the pistol back into my pack, and stepped out from behind the rock. Dolma stopped and looked at me, half-smiled, and said, "Did everything go all right?"

I did not respond directly. "I spent the night here. They must still be up ahead of us."

"Well, I guess you must have done all right. I found this along the trail." He opened his hand to show me the object he had been jiggling in his palm. It was the brass-bright casing of a 45 slug. "How many did you get?"

"There was only the one. He had a radio. But no one else has come."

"Yes, there was probably only the one," Dolma shook his head in agreement. "By the way, I broke down the assault rifle and put it in the pony's pack. Figured since you left it behind, I could use it."

"You can keep it."

103

"What about the pistol? If you don't want it, I could use that, too."

"Tell you what, Dolma. I'll give it to you when we get back to Pokhara. Just in case."

"Yes, just in case. Good choice." And he looked at me in a different way.

I changed the subject. "Did you have any trouble coming up over the Thapa La behind me, or anything else?"

"Well, some friends of mine in Baglung told me you had passed through, and that the weather had been good, but that there was a big early snow going to come in over the Thapa La the next night. So I took a chance and circled back and came right up the Kali Ghandaki, right through the gorge, along the east bank, as clear as could be. Nobody paid any attention to one dumb Bhoti leading a single pony, probably thought I was headed up to Mustang to smuggle a few bolts of cloth or a bottle of whiskey across into Tibet. I forded the Kali at that place below Jomosom, into Marpha. Nobody paid any attention there either, even if this Bhoti did spend three years at Texas A and M."

Despite myself, I grinned. "Damn, I *knew* there was something about your accent."

We decided to keep moving up the trail, in case our party was in some kind of difficulty. I lashed my backpack on the top of the pony's packsaddle. But I took out the pistol, cleared the chamber, and stashed it in my pocket.

We kept moving for several hours, without speaking, on a trail that moved higher and higher into the desolate mountains. The trail was faint, and seemed little used. We saw no villages, and passed no travelers, along the way.

Dolma was in front, leading the pony. I brought up the rear. Abruptly, he stopped and raised a nail-grimed finger towards a distant ridge.

"Here they come."

6

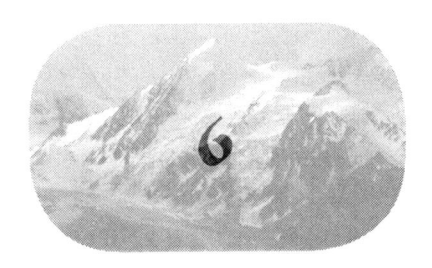

We stood and watched them approach. As the figures came nearer, we could make them out more clearly. There were two, in Tibetan robes, walking in front. In the rear were two more, one in the robes of a monk and leading a lightly-packed yak. In the middle was a figure riding a yak. As they got closer still, we could see that there was something wrong with the rider, who was also dressed as a monk. He was stretched forward, laid out along the yak's neck, and he looked as if he was tied into the packsaddle. He rolled from side to side, in passive response, as the animal moved along on a short lead held by one of the figures in front.

The travelers could now see us. One pointed, and assumed a wary posture. I could see now that the two in front were armed, with what appeared to be similar short assault rifles as the one I had taken from the Young Chinese Soldier.

They stopped, a hundred yards or so from us, and then one of those in front gave a shout of recognition and rushed on toward us.

"Dolma, is all well with you? Still you are stealing whiskey and chasing women?"

"Yes, Tsing-Ba, unlike you I am more Bon than Buddhist. It is good to see you, even if you speak bad English instead of good Tibetan. This is Doctor Joseph. He speaks English, too." Two others ran up, bursting into Tibetan. The walking monk came on slowly, now leading both the yaks, one carrying the pack, and the other burdened with the rider.

The travelers and Dolma embraced. There were more torrents of Tibetan. My eyes were on the figure tied into the saddle of the yak.

Dolma turned to me. "They have had a very hard time crossing the Pindu La, though they have seen no Chinese soldiers since leaving

Lhasa many days ago. The boy, whom they are transporting, is very ill."

"Let's get him off the yak, and let me have a look at him. How long has he been sick?"

Tsing-Ba, whose English was not quite as good as Dolma's, said, "Three days, maybe four. It was hard difficult crossing the *La* with him in this way, two days ago. He is a good boy, and tries not to complain, but he is not a Khamba, not a soldier. He is a monk. He has bad pains in his middle, and was vomiting all times until today morning. No shit, little piss. We have tried to give him as much water, but he takes only some little. He seems hot, then cold. It was very bad for him, on the yak, but what could we do? It was very cold, and we were all of us afraid, for him and for ourselves as well. I think he must die."

Laid out on a wool blanket on the ground, the boy, who appeared to be about thirteen, was semiconscious. He resisted being straightened in the supine position, tried to curl himself to the right, turning half on his side. He was pale and gray, warm but not with a raging fever. Thin bilious spittle was caked on his chin, and his robe was stained with vomit. His eyes were sunken from dehydration. He mumbled a few words, which I could not make out, and when I tried to meet his eyes I could read no expression in them. The boy had been very ill for days now, was desperately ill, but alone in his pain, looking only inside himself, and expecting neither help nor relief.

I parted his robe, and examined his belly. He was thin, but the muscles of his belly were board-rigid. His most sensitive point seemed to be low along the right side of his abdomen, slightly over toward his belly-button. When I pushed firmly on his abdominal muscles, anywhere, and let go quickly, he moaned and reached feebly for that one most painful location, the one that we learn early in medical school is called "McBurney's Point."

Without taking the time to search in my pack for a rubber glove, I inserted my index finger into his rectum. It was empty. When I pressed against the rectal wall on his left side, he fidgeted irritably. When I pressed against the wall on the right side, he whined in pain, like a badly injured dog.

I wiped my finger on his robe, and stepped back. The Tibetans were looking at me.

Every third-year med student knows what this is, and every first-year surgical resident knows how to fix it. But goddamn it, I'm up here on the Tibetan border with five guys, three of whom don't speak English, and all I have is what's in my pack, and I'm not a surgeon, and I've seen this done but have never done it by myself.

I was alone and afraid.

I turned to Dolma. "This boy has, I am very sure, an acute appendix. You know what that means?" Dolma nodded, expressionless, and I continued. "His appendix may have already ruptured, broken open into the belly cavity, but I don't think so, but I can't be sure. At any rate, it is probably slowly leaking pus into his belly as we speak. If that continues, or the appendix ruptures, he will have peritonitis, and die of the poisoning. He is very dehydrated from the vomiting, and not drinking, and being at these high altitudes, and in poor general condition. He will die if he is not operated on, and soon."

Tsing-Ba, who was following as best he could, said, "How can we take him all the way to Shining Hospital, four or five days? There is nowhere else."

"We can't," I replied. "He would never last, even if it wasn't for the difficulty of the travel. We fix him, close to here, or he dies. If he is your special Lama, we must try, as soon as possible."

The Tibetans shuffled their feet, and Dolma looked at me, half-defiantly and half-sheepishly. "Steve, there is something you don't know, but now must know. This boy, who is called Pemba, is not the Lama. We brought him down as a decoy for the Chinese. The real Incarnate Lama came down through the east, way over by Chainpur, down the Arun Khola valley. He is now safe in Darjeeling, and the Indians will take good care of him, since they have been given plenty of rupees to do so. Soon he will go by train to meet with His Holiness, the Dalai Lama, at Dharamsala. I got this word before I left Pokhara; that is why I was waiting and came up after you did. What I am saying, Steve, is that this is a boy of little signficance."

My mind whirled with a combination of anger and guilt: anger at the Tibetans' deception of me and their callous use of the boy as a pawn, and guilt at my own actions in consequence of that deception.

"Damn you for a treacherous son of a bitch, Dolma! Goddamndamn you. You mean that all of this was a charade? Me coming up here, going around the back way, meeting the Chinese . . . " I had to stop, could go no further.

"Steve, hear me. We have been betrayed so many times, for so long. We can trust no one. You must see that it was an important ruse. The Chinese did in fact try to stop this caravan, and blocked the major passes in the Center, while we were able to sneak the real Lama out through the East. I am not sorry to lie to you, my friend. I will do whatever I have to do for my people."

"Well, who knew? Was Bill Thompson part of the ruse? Did my Embassy know this was all a fake? Who knew that this boy was, as you so-casually put it, "of little significance?""

"I do not know who knew what. I am a soldier and I do what I am told. But now you tell me, what do we do?"

I thought for a moment. "We will go back down to Marpha. There is an abandoned Nepali government health post there. We will try to keep him alive until we get to Marpha. Then we will do what we need to do, and hope that we can do enough."

Before we started down toward Marpha, I soaked a rag in water from a canteen, and pushed the rag's end into a corner of Pemba's mouth. Through Dolma, I told the monk to keep the rag moistened, but not to put so much water on it that it would choke him, and not to stuff the rag into his mouth so far that it would make his breathing more difficult.

He was very weak, but I thought that the boy understood a little of what was going on around him, and certainly he was aware of his pain. The motion of the yak on the stony trail must have been agony for him, but the broader platform of the yak's back was probably easier on him than sitting in a pony's saddle would have been. I gave him fifty milligrams of Demerol by mouth to help the pain, and that seemed to ease him some, but I was worried about over-sedating him in his weakened condition. That would pose a great problem when we got to Marpha, and I had to anesthetize him as best I could for surgery. Too much? Too little? It was a dilemma that weighed on my mind.

We moved out in single file, sending one of the Khambas as a runner ahead. His instructions from Dolma were to make sure that there were no Chinese back along the trail, no police or soldiers in Marpha, and that the Nepali Health Post was not occupied. He was then to move quickly back up the trail and meet us on the way in.

I judged that it would take us about five hours' travel to reach Marpha. Since it was now about nine in the morning, we should arrive there about two in the afternoon.

I used the time on the trail to work out for myself, over and over again in my mind, what needed to be done, and what I had and didn't have, and what could be done with what I had, however inadequately prepared and supplied I might be.

It is a general rule in medicine that whenever you have obstruction in a non-sterile environment, you will sooner or later have infection. The entire digestive tract can be thought of as a hollow tube, open at each end, sitting *within* the other tube formed by the internal cavities of the body. While the chest and abdominal cavities themselves are, and need to remain, sterile, the digestive tube, which in a certain sense is *outside* the body, is anything but sterile. It is full of bacteria and other micro-organisms, which must be prevented from reaching the bloodstream or the body cavities. Thus, when the appendix, a blind-ended narrow pouch coming off the main intestinal channel, becomes obstructed, inflamed, and infected, the symptoms of acute appendicitis appear. The abscess that forms can seep, or burst, into the abdominal cavity itself. The medical word for the infection of the abdominal cavity that follows is *peritonitis*, and it is highly likely to be fatal once it takes hold, unless treated intensively with measures that I did not have at my disposal. So, the only preventive medicine and the only therapy for this inflamed appendix was to remove it surgically. Even that might prove too late if the appendix had already ruptured and significant peritonitis had set in. There was essentially zero chance of keeping this patient alive during a three- or four- day rough journey by yak over uneven trails to reach the nearest hospital and surgeons, at the Shining Hospital in Pokhara.

I was quite confident of my trailside diagnosis in this case, but there are, unfortunately, many other surgical and medical conditions which the unwary, unskilled, or unlucky may mistakenly diagnose as acute appendicitis. I could not help but think of how much easier it would have sounded, amidst the technical comforts and supports of an American hospital, to hear the old saying, "When it doubt, take it out." First year surgical residents learn to do appendectomies in their sleep. It is considered the least complicated of abdominal emergency operations, and they have first assistants, scrub nurses, circulating nurses, anesthetists, and senior physicians to help and guide them, and laboratory tests pre-operatively to help confirm the diagnosis, or to point in other directions. It would be quite different in Marpha.

Thinking about the support system back home under those bright lights of the operating room, I was suddenly aware of what might prove to be the undoing of my plans. There was a critical factor that is usually taken for granted.

Light! If we arrived in Marpha about two in the afternoon, and it took me an hour to get organized, it would be, say, three p.m. before I could begin surgery. Dark comes early to the Himalayas in September. There was no electricity within three days' walk. I would have to arrange for the Tibetans, with whatever flashlights and lanterns we would be able to muster, to give me light down in that dark hole in the belly. I urged Dolma, "We must go faster," and then realized that if I pushed the yak too fast, I might not have a live patient when we arrived in Marpha. I thought back about all those times in my life when I had unthinkingly pushed a switch, and was annoyed if the light bulb was blown, or arranged a goose-neck lamp for my comfort or convenience, or heard someone tell me as a child not to "strain my eyes" when reading "without proper light."

About an hour out of Marpha, we met the returning Tibetan runner.

Dolma questioned him closely, and then turned to me.

"He says that he is confident that the coast is clear ahead. Further, he has located a friend (probably a confederate smuggler) in Marpha who can be counted on to help us in any way we need. It is safe to push on."

The government health post was situated, off by itself, to the north of the village. With its peeling whitewash, and its sagging roof, it was distinguished by the red cross painted on the building, which was a two-room mud and wattle structure. The windows were grimy, and the lock on the door gave easily to Dolma's shoulder. The larger room held a concrete counter and sink, and a wooden examining table. In the second room, there were two wooden chairs and a number of equipment and dispensary cabinets, doors hanging partly open and askew.

Apart from that, the health post was completely, and utterly, empty. Not a basin, not a bandage, not a piece of paper. The only other things besides the bare walls were the dried pellets left by some small animal in one corner.

For the moment, I had the Tibetans make up a pallet with blankets along one wall for the boy. His pulse was rapid, but regular and not too weak. He seemed eager to suck on his cloth, but in great pain, and sweaty and restless in his semi-conscious state. I did not want to give him any further medication until we actually prepared for surgery.

One of the Khambas went off into the village, and shortly reappeared with two Thakalis, an old man and a younger one. Dolma put a hand on one shoulder of each of the newcomers, rattled off a string of Tibetan at them, and then translated for me what he had said to them: "I am glad that you are our friends and will help us. After we finish here, you must take us into your house, and feed and hide us. When we are able to leave Marpha, if all has gone well, we will leave for you the two yaks as a present. But if we are betrayed, or found by any Nepali or Chinese soldiers, I will shoot the two yaks first, and then I will shoot you."

The Thakalis seemed to have gotten the message. I saw them speaking to each other outside, standing beside the immeasurably-valuable yaks, stroking their flanks, and then leading the yaks and the pony away. I realized that they would be unlikely to have much love for any Nepali government officials and would have none at all for the Chinese. If we got through the next few hours successfully, we were probably safe in the village for the several days needed for the boy's convalescence, unless some chance occurrence, or some individual's greed, gave us away.

"Dolma," I said. "You must find the following things quickly. Send Tsing-Ba and the other two Khambas to his friend's house and to other houses for these things. You and I and the monk will start by cleaning up this place as best we can, using water from our canteens and rags torn from clothing and blankets. We must clean the windows well, and let in all the light we can. Here are the things I need: water in large jugs; several pots with covers; three or four metal spoons, as large as you can find, and they must be metal, not wooden; wood and charcoal for making a fire in that sink; a lantern or two. And bring some *rakshi*, which you must not drink. Hurry."

While Dolma and the monk finished washing down the table and the counter, and cleaning the windows, I went through my medical kit, without opening anything that was sealed, and took stock of what I had.

There were several things that I knew I did not have. I had neither intravenous fluids nor the means of infusing them. I had no blood to transfuse. If the boy went into shock or if my clumsy and untrained fingers cut a vessel that I couldn't clamp and tie, we were out of luck. I had no oxygen, and no ether or other inhalation anesthetic. Good anesthesia is important, not only for pain relief, but also for relaxing the spasm of the abdominal wall muscles so that I could work more easily. I would just have to do without these things.

And if the appendix had already burst, or if I burst it or allowed it to spill its contents during the surgery, the boy would almost certainly die.

I found that I had only three packets of sterile surgical gloves, and I knew that everything might depend on keeping the surgical field as sterile as possible. I was also dangerously short of surgical clamps. The best I could do was two fair-sized hemostats, one alligator clamp, and a small mosquito clamp. I would need everything I had for clamping off bleeding vessels, and for double-clamping the appendix before I tied off the stump and cut it loose.

The scavenging expedition returned, well-stocked, and sooner that I had expected. I began to lay out my plan, and the materials I would need, explaining to Dolma each step as I went along, and having him translate into Tibetan for the others.

We took my ground cloth, which we had washed down as well as possible, and cut it in half. One half was laid on the wooden table, which would be our operating site. We moved the table near, and perpendicular to, the concrete counter. On half of the long counter, well away from the sink, we placed the other half of the ground cloth. On the other half of the counter, we placed the four or five pots and basins. We built a fire in the sink, and used the largest basin to boil water, pouring the water from repeated boilings into the set-aside pots and smaller basins. Then we gently lifted the boy, and laid him on the ground cloth, which covered what I now thought of as the operating table, arranging his clothing so that he was naked and exposed from his breastbone to below his groin.

At one end of the covered counter, I placed those things that I would need but which would remain unsterile: a Sierra cup full of water, and gauze with which to drip a little liquid into the boy's mouth; a three-ounce bottle of sterile novocaine solution, its rubber cap swabbed with an alcohol sponge; a bottle containing iodoform gauze wick (with the screw cap undone but left loosely in place).

I took all three paper-wrapped packets of sterile surgical gloves and tore them open, as one would open a book, but I did not reach into the inner packets which protected the gloves themselves. I laid all three opened packets on the other half of the ground cloth, which was now to define my sterile supply area. I opened, without touching the contents, the metal-paper or plastic coverings that housed the following equipment, and dropped the equipment carefully on top of two of the three sterile opened glove packets: several disposable syringes of various sizes, a larger number of disposable needles which would fit on the hubs of the syringes, a scalpel handle and a few scalpel blades, several packets of suture material, a selection of sterile gauze squares and a roll of gauze bandage.

I set two final pots of water to boiling, and dumped into one of them what were to be my sterile instruments: all the clamps and forceps, a pair of surgical scissors, and the four long metal spoons that the Tibetans had scrounged. Before putting them on the boil, I had bent the ends of each of the spoons, about three or four inches from the handle's end, so that they formed a right angle. These were to serve as the retractors that would hold open the edges of the surgical incision while I worked.

Between me and the Tibetans, we had four fairly serviceable

flashlights, and the very bright but small-field light of my otoscope. I was for once thankful that my obsessive-compulsive personality had led me to carry all this various stuff around, many times cursing at its weight and volume in my pack.

I explained, through Dolma's interpretation, what everyone was to do. "Dolma, you are my Surgical Assistant. You will have on only one single glove, on your right hand. You will pass me the sterilized things that I ask for, and take back the things I am finished with, with only that one hand. You must touch nothing else in the operating field or in the sterile area of the counter unless I specifically tell you to. In your other, "unclean" left hand, you hold this flashlight in case we need extra illumination. You two, you Khamba warriors, you will each also have only one glove on. Your jobs are to stand one on each side of the table. You will each have one flashlight in your ungloved hand, and in your other, clean and gloved, hand you will have one of the bent spoons, after I place it and tell you to take it from me. It will be used like a hook, to hold the edges of the open wound apart, so I can work deep in the belly."

As Dolma translated, the Khambas nodded slowly, impassively.

"You must pull hard, and hold steady, like you are pulling the lead rope on a stubborn yak. It will be hard work, but you are strong, and I know I can count on you not to let go.

"Tsing-Ba. You will stand on the opposite side of the table from Dolma and me. You will have no gloves, but you will hold this bright small light, and shine it exactly where I tell you into the wound.

"And you, Monk, you will stand in the corner over there, watch that the boy still breathes, and be ready to do whatever we need to help us if a problem arises. And, you can pray for us and this boy.

"Remember, all of you, that neither you nor your clothing is allowed to touch anything that we consider clean. Be careful if you have to lean over the boy. I know that the Tibetans have a saying about foreigners (outside men) and Tibetans (inside men): The outside man is clean outside; the inside man is clean inside. But I know that you are Khambas, and that you are clean both outside and inside. So let us, together, save the life of this boy, even if he is of 'little significance,' as are we all."

The Tibetans nodded and mumbled as Dolma gave them the instructions. There were neither questions nor comments. I was proud to work with them, these soldier/bandit/smuggler patriots of a country that no one seemed to care about, except for those rosy idealists in safe places who dared do nothing nasty to make the world what they wished it would be. And so, we began.

My professors of anesthesiology would not be pleased by how I began. As surgeons did before the modern age of anesthesia, I administered small sips of the *rakshi* liquor, almost drop by drop so that the boy would not choke on it. My end point was when the boy began to snore, and then I gave him a little more, for good measure.

Next, I opened the little plastic box in which I carried what I considered my emergency medications. I dropped a glass vial of morphine onto the non-sterile section of the supply counter, followed by a vial of adrenaline and one of calcium solution. The latter two were for last-ditch use in case the patient's heart stopped. In for a penny, in for a pound.

"You, Monk, pick up this vial of morphine. Touch nothing else. Hold it by the bottom end." This, as with everything else, had to go through Dolma for translation. I used my unsterile hand to snap off the top of the vial, then took a small syringe, fitted on to it a small gauge needle (now only the needle was sterile, as it had come out of its sheath untouched by my hands). I drew up 10 milligrams of morphine, no, shot the moon for 15 milligrams, and injected it into the boy's shoulder muscle. I accompanied this with an irreverent prayer that the morphine and *rakshi* would not depress my weakened patient's respiration beyond some point of no return. So far, so good; he fell deeply asleep, breathing regularly and not too shallowly, not too deeply.

I scrubbed my hands with soap and hot water, and then, though my hands were by no means truly sterile, I used hot water and soap to scrub the boy's abdomen, following up by using the few iodine-soaked small pads I had in my medical kit to sanitize the lower abdomen on the right side. Employing the same procedure as previously with the assistance of the monk, I injected a line of novocaine beneath the skin where I planned to make my incision.

Now came the hard part. I scrubbed my hands and forearms for a second time with soap, as vigorously as I could in one of the pots of water as hot as I could take it, and had the others do the same. We shook our hands in the air, and waited impatiently until they dried, each alone with our thoughts.

I looked at Dolma. We locked eyes and held each other's gaze. Then Dolma broke contact and looked down at the floor.

Cautiously, I lifted open the one package of sterile gloves that had not been covered with sterile equipment, and put on the gloves. I had Dolma transmit to the others the specific instructions for doing likewise with their single gloves. Then I shifted the sterile equipment that had been dropped on the other two sterile opened packets onto the one packet, still relatively sterile, that I had just emptied. Using my sterile gloved hands, I lifted open the two remaining sterile packets, and had Dolma and the two Khambas each put on a glove on a right hand. This left only one sterile glove as a back-up in case I contaminated myself and needed to change a glove.

The process would not pass muster at the Massachusetts General Hospital, but it went fairly well, and the Tibetans proved quite dexterous, as do many people who do not have the distractions of omnipresent machinery to dull their tactile abilities. I debated with myself as to whether I should now change my right glove for the one sterile glove remaining, and decided, no, it would be better to leave it in reserve, as a back up in case of real emergency.

Before going further, I had the two Khambas and Tsing-Ba focus their flashlights, held in their ungloved hands, on the general area where I was going to work. All to this point was preparation. I now had my semi-sterile gloves, a semi-sterile environment, and could pick up, or have Dolma hand to me, the sterile equipment resting on the semi-sterile paper packet supply area and get on with it.

Surgeons pride themselves on making the smallest and neatest incision possible. That would have been foolish in my case. I needed a big hole to let inadequate light and clumsy fingers in. I fitted a scalpel blade to the metal handle, and cut a generous line through the skin and subcutaneous tissue in the right lower quadrant of the abdomen, parallel and fairly close above the bone that forms the forward upper edge of the pelvic basin. There were a few small bleeders, nothing more.

God looks after kids and ill-trained surgeons, at least in some cases.

I had Dolma hand me the mosquito clamp, and at times one or both hemostats, with his gloved hand. I clamped off each bleeding vessel, and then I tied off each one individually by myself, which took more time than when you have a First Assistant to hold the clamp and cut the ends off the knots as you finish tying them.

Now I was down to cutting through the layers of muscle. The spasm was only partially relaxed, but enough so that I could proceed. I dared not look up at the boy's face, just let my inner mind listen to the rhythm of his breathing. Occasionally I flicked my eyes upwards to watch the motion of his chest, while trying not to lose my focus of concentration on the abdomen. There were some more bleeders, only one of which was of worrisome size, and I dealt with them as I had the others. I cut through the glistening peritoneal layer concealing the abdominal cavity itself. I thought of Old Tommy Grendlen, my professor of surgery, who was a real knuckle-knocker, employing a steel forceps to punish a medical student's clumsy knot tying. "Tommy—why ain't you here now to show me how to really do it," I muttered to myself. Dolma duly translated, and the other Tibetans looked puzzled.

Then, using the same scissors I had employed to cut the suture knots, which would have gotten me tossed out of any American operating room, I cut several long strips of the sterile gauze, placed them in the margins of the wound, and then placed the improvised wound retractors where they would do the most good. Dolma was proving himself to be an excellent scrub nurse, giving and receiving instruments crisply with his single gloved hand, dropping the used ones back on the sterile paper for further use.

"Here, hang on to these, and don't you dare ease up," I said to the two Khambas, handing over the retractors, one to each of them in a gloved hand. I thought again of medical student days, hanging on to those retractors for what seemed hours on end, trying to stay awake at the same time, knees ready to give out, hemorrhoids developing nicely, and Old Tommy and his ilk ready to pop you a good one if your pressure on the retractor was not strong and, above all, steady.

"May these guys be better than I was," I said. They were.

Okay so far, now we were down to the real business. There before me, reflected in the focused light of Tsing-Ba's otoscope, were the glistening shiny loops of small bowel, squirming slowly like eels. No signs of generalized infection, no pus in the abdominal cavity that I could see at first glance.

I took a deep breath, had Dolma hand me several sterile gauze squares, and as gently as I could, scooped the small bowel to one side, digging down in that lower right quadrant. There she was— a tiny bloated sausage, with a purplish greenish yellowish hue, just a hint of pus maybe at one side, but basically intact. So the Fates were still with us. No troubles with an appendix tucked back up under and behind the large intestine. No burst balloon. No pus on the loose. No peritonitis. Easy money, provided I could handle the basics.

I took another cut length of sterile gauze to hold the small bowel aside, and had Dolma hand me the two hemostats. I double-clamped the appendix, placing the two hemostats very closely together. Then I tied a suture, just as tight as I could get it, close to the base of the swollen appendix, and another suture on the far side of the second clamp. So, starting at the point where the appendix came off of the intestine, I had *suture, clamp, clamp, suture.* Then I took a deep breath, and, using the scalpel, cut off the appendix between the two clamps. I guess I expected a thunderclap or something, but nothing happened. My hands shaking slightly, I lifted the appendix from the abdomen and dropped it onto the unsterile part of the counter, unclamping the hemostat for further emergency use if need be, though I would have to consider it now grossly contaminated. Then I unclamped the other hemostat, the one on the tied-off business end of the appendiceal stump, very carefully, and tried as best I could to perform the suturing process of inverting the stump. I did a quite poor job of that, but at least it held.

I don't remember very clearly my journey out of the belly, closing each tissue layer one after the other with sutures. I left a small gap at the lower end of the wound, and used the alligator forceps to push in a length of iodoform gauze. I had the monk hold up the bottle by its lower end, and shake off the loosened cap without touching the bottle top itself; then I reached in and pulled out the iodoform gauze strip with the forceps, and cut off a length with the scissors. The iodine-impregnated gauze strip would serve as a wick to drain the wound, and would be pulled out, just like the one in the drained thigh abscess in the PCV at Baglung, three or so days later. The final skin layer was closed, a retention stitch put into the skin to hold the wick in place, and I used a loose dressing made of the sterile gauze squares.

It was done. Dolma told me later that the process, from skin to skin, took about sixty minutes. A good surgical team can probably do it in fifteen or twenty, much more safely, and with a prettier result. If any real surgeon was to look at that scar, or go back in the belly a few years later, he would only shake his head and cluck like a chicken at the thought of the barber who had done that job.

Only then did I ask the monk, "Does he still breathe?"

"The boy lives," he replied.

"For now," was my rejoinder, and I noticed that my hands were shaking, and that the shivering had spread to my arms and legs.

I just stood and watched him for a while. His color was terrible, but his breathing was steady. The Tibetans were all still standing at their stations, waiting for what came next, whether from me or from the patient.

After a bit, I said, "Let's clean up. Thank you. You did well. Thank you."

Then I told Dolma what to do in the next hours: "Watch the boy, look for any bleeding around the wound, check his breathing and pulse, try to give him small drips of water through a mouth cloth, see if his skin gets hot, or cold, or clammy." The Khambas had seen enough wounded and dying, surely many more than I had, and they knew pretty much what to do.

I decided against giving any more sedation or painkillers for the present, but just to let his body do its work for him. I did give him a shot of about half the long-acting injectable antibiotics that I had, according to the old "just in case" principle, which I had been taught in medical school was the wrong thing to do. But this was Marpha, not medical school, and I had enough injectables left for another shot in twelve hours, and then pills that would last another two or three days.

I watched him some more for what seemed a long time, a time without time, like that in the river. Then weariness overcame me. I let myself sink onto my knees at the side of the table, and laid my head next to the boy's chest.

And I wept. I wept for this boy "of little significance." I wept for the Young Chinese Soldier. And most of all I wept for myself, for borders that had been crossed and could never again be crossed in the opposite direction. I wept until no more tears would come, and then I slept.

When I awoke, I found that the Tibetans had laid me on one blanket, and covered me with another. The light seemed to be that of midday, so surely many hours of a night and a morning had passed. I turned my head, and in the other corner, half sitting, was the Tibetan boy. Pemba saw my opened eyes, and smiled, and, believe it or not, he gave me a thumbs-up. Beside him was a small brass cup, from which Tsing-Ba was giving him sips of water or perhaps of rice broth. He would live.

That day we moved into the house at the end of the village. We carried Pemba, who said little but smiled often, in a blanket litter. We stayed in that house for six days. The wick drain came out, clean as a whistle, on the third day.

After I pulled the drain, I walked out of Marpha, back along the trail I had originally come on, back towards the Thapa La. I had some hope of seeing the magic of the pass again. But there was snow now as the trail rose, and cold biting wind, and I turned back to the village, hunched over against the wind, after only a little distance.

In a week Pemba was clearly strong and well-healed enough to travel. We put him on the pony, and forded the river at night, over to the east bank, unseen by anyone but the Marpha villagers. We camped right alongside the trail, well into the Kali Ghandaki gorge, and on the first full day of travel, Pemba walked for an hour or so, and rode the rest. By the third day, after we had passed Tatopani, he walked the entire time. We saw few travelers, none of whom showed much interest in us. We saw no police, and no soldiers. We spoke little among ourselves, and the pony bells were the sound that we heard most of.

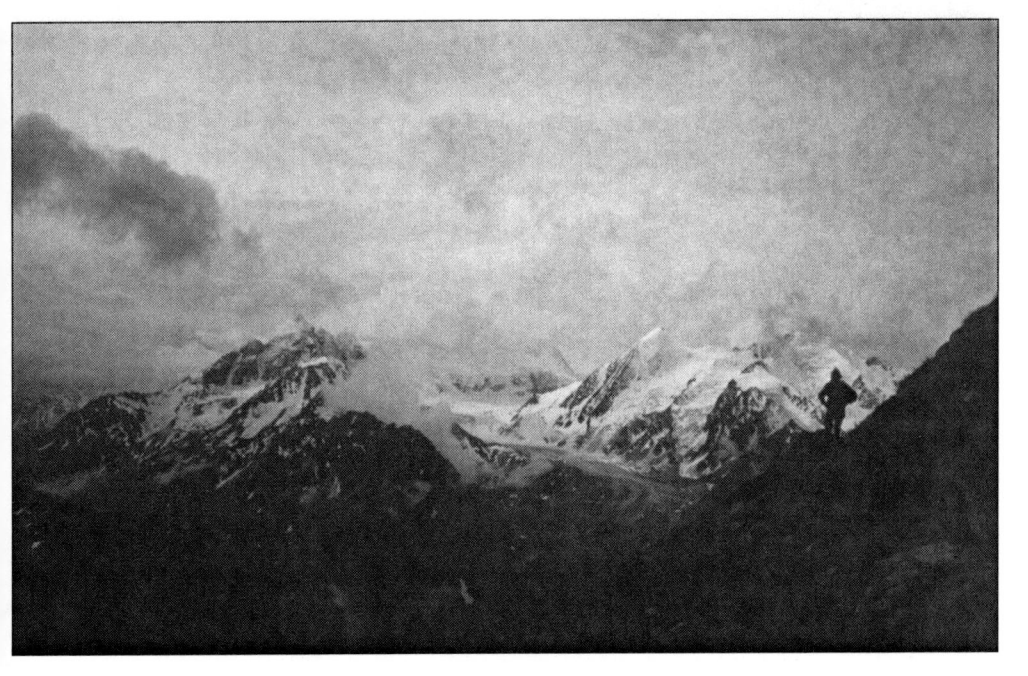

River of stone

One of the Khambas had moved swiftly ahead of us on the fourth and last day coming down from Marpha, and when we reached the Tibetan refugee camp outside of Pokhara there was a small silent crowd awaiting us. I saw the young woman who had been rolling bandages that first day I came to the camp step forward and gently put her hand on Dolma's shoulder.

I sought out the Italian doctor. "You son of a bitch, you knew I was on a fool's errand," I said, but I smiled as I said it. I returned his sweater, now grimy and greasy, and told him I would repay him a pound of rice the next time I came by.

It was hard to say goodbye to Dolma, Tsing-Ba, the others, and to Pemba. Dolma said, "It has been good to walk the trail with you. Forgive my lies, or at least understand the reasons for them."

"There is nothing to forgive, Dolma," I replied. "As you say, you are a soldier and do what you are told."

Pemba, standing straight in his monk's robe, said nothing, but put his palm upon my forehead.

Tsing-Ba, of all people, gave me a small brown and white Tibetan woven wool rug. I tied it on top of my pack. It still sits at the foot of my bed, and always will.

When I got back to Kathmandu, it took me several days to sort out all the things that had gone on in my absence.

On the second day, Harry Barkely phoned from the Embassy.

"Welcome back, Steve. The Ambassador would like you to drop by so I can have a few words with you."

I caught the innuendo. Not "The Ambassador wants to see you," but a layer interposed between him and myself. Smoothly done.

Harry was as relaxed as ever in his small office.

"Uh, Steve, have some more coffee? We've been hearing some minor rumbles from His Majesty's Government, about some kind or other of difficulties up beyond Jomosom. I hope you didn't exceed your instructions and go further north toward the Tibetan frontier. Was there some kind of misunderstanding as to what you and your friend Bill Thompson were supposed to be doing?"

I caught the emphasis on "your friend".

"Harry, there is always the possibility of misunderstanding when someone is cut out of the loop as to what is really going on."

"Hmm." Harry kept that bland, or rather blank, stare that diplomats affect when they want to close off a discussion without giving anything further away. But I thought I could see just the slightest clenching of his jaw muscles, just the least little bit. Was it possible that he didn't know himself? Or was he passing on a message from above: "Keep your mouth shut about what never happened."

"Well, in the future be more careful. And perhaps you ought to avoid that area for a while. That's what the Ambassador wanted me to tell you."

Willi was somewhat more direct, but equally ambiguous.

"Holy Cow, Steve, what the heck did you get into up there? Your buddy Thompson blew in and out of town here without even dropping by the Office to leave any word of your trip together. Well, good riddance to him. Florence put him in a walking cast and he hobbled out on the next day's plane. It's all a mystery to me. I'm glad it was in no way Peace Corps business."

"Well, Willi, not to concern yourself. All our people are all right in the region. The usual minor medical stuff. This and that and a bit of the other. Just took somewhat longer than I had expected."

I never did really know who knew how much about what had happened, or had a hand in setting the wheels in motion. No one in the Embassy, or at the Peace Corps office, ever asked me anything more about it.

When my two-year tour was up, I returned to Boston and to my pediatric residency. I still loved my work, but there was a spark gone out of it for me, or perhaps more accurately, a spark gone out of me, or perhaps even a spark burning in a different place within me. I found it difficult to translate to my colleagues what the two years had been about, and learned painfully that their interest expired after a few perfunctory questions. It was easier, I decided, to try and fit in with their world, at least for the present, to immerse myself in their busy world of big-city academic U.S. pediatrics.

But I was restless, and knew that there was now a place within me that I would not share with others, and most of the time would not share with myself. The Young Chinese Soldier came often into my dreams, more often than Pemba or Dolma, or the others.

I sometimes wondered what had become of Bill Thompson. Had he gone to Vietnam, had he come back, how had it changed him? What could he have known about what happened up north, unless Dolma was even more than he had seemed, and there was some back-channel to the Embassy in Kathmandu?

Harry Barkely had a long and distinguished Foreign Service Career, achieving Ambassadorial rank. We remained friends, at a distance, and there were many things we never talked about.

Ambassador Stubblefield disappeared, presumably overboard,

during a Trans-Atlantic ocean passage on his trip home to the States at the end of his tour in Nepal. No body was ever found.

Willi died on the mountain, younger than he should have, but in a manner that I believe he would have chosen, leading a group of students to safety off Mount Rainier in a storm, overtaken by an avalanche.

Dolma and Pemba, and the rest, wherever they are, are still waiting for their country's freedom.

PART TWO

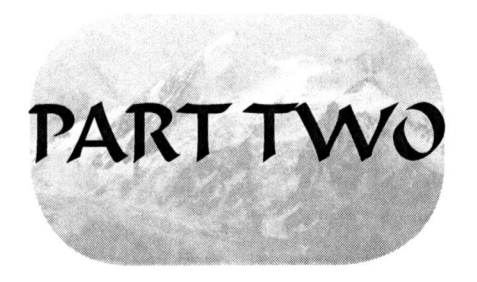

RIVER OF SAND
WEST AFRICA, 1970–1973

Epidemic: From the Greek; *epi*= upon, *demos*= the people

7

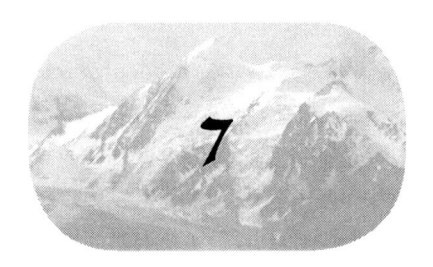

The next three or four years, following my return from Nepal, passed slowly. I felt not so much that I was marking time, but that I was running furiously in place. There were personal and professional achievements and satisfactions, but when you added it all up, I felt empty, unfed. Or rather, fed to overfilling, but unsatisfied.

During the last months of my tour in Nepal, on an occasion when I was back in Washington with a medical evacuation, I had been asked to meet with a Public Health Service recruiter. This doctor, who had himself recently returned from a year in Vietnam, asked if I would accept an assignment in Saigon, part of a PHS group working to upgrade a civilian hospital. I thought about it for several minutes. My eyes kept coming back to what seemed to me to be an incongruous paperweight on his desk, an inactivated hand grenade. The Young Chinese Soldier whispered in my ear, "Who are you to judge?"

I thought through all the reasons that would argue for me declining. I had a growing young family. My marriage was under strain, and I doubted it could survive a year's absence in Saigon. I was anxious to get on with my specialty training in pediatrics. I had just been in Asia for two years. I was confused and uncertain about how I felt personally about the war, uneasy that the arguments my government was making just didn't seem to add up. Yet I understood the enormous sacrifices that were being made by individuals in the war's prosecution, most of them individuals who had very little choice over their actions, many of them better men than I would ever be. All the usual stuff one tells oneself. And I thought less of myself, and still do, for turning him down.

That feeling strengthened in me a year or two later, when a best friend of my childhood, Peter Worthington, deployed to Vietnam as an Army psychiatrist. By a series of strange coincidences, Peter and I had spent kindergarten, first grade, high school, a year of college, and all of medical school together. We had been close, and Peter was, even more than I was, something of a natural outsider. He had chosen psychiatry, and opted for the "Berry Plan," by which the military allowed him to finish his civilian residency, and then took him into the Army as a specialist in his field. When he went to Vietnam, he left at home a wife and an infant son, both of whom he adored.

Peter hated the war. He was posted as far forward as psychiatrists got, and his letters home talked of how he felt about figuratively patching up kids so that they could go back into the line.

Halfway through his tour, Peter's wife, Syble, was supposed to come with Oliver, now almost two years old, and spend Thanksgiving with my family and me. At the last moment she telephoned, filled with excitement. Peter had cabled that he could get a week's leave and a flight out, and could she and Oliver meet him in Hawaii? When they arrived by commercial air at the Honolulu airport, on Thanksgiving Day, they were met on the tarmac not by Peter, but by the casualty officer. The helicopter carrying Captain Worthington had been shot down upon take-off from his jungle airstrip for the short hop to Danang. There was one survivor, but it was not Peter.

So why him and not me, I thought. Why does one go this way, and one go the other way?

As for the way I went, the Public Health Service had offered me a place in a new training program, aimed at preparing young physicians for public health and community medicine in both the U.S. and overseas. So I kept my commission, stayed on active duty with PHS for a total of five years, got pediatric and public health credentials, and then sort of drifted into technical and administrative medical roles with the Federal Government.

It was useful, maybe even important, work, building and overseeing the development of neighborhood health centers in poor urban and rural communities. But I had the clear understanding that I was becoming less of a doctor and more of a suit. Although I moonlighted in hospital emergency rooms to keep my hand in and my experience growing, I knew that I was turning further and further away from my Shining Mountains.

Two other former Peace Corps docs and myself talked about going in together and starting a model rural private practice, based on the health center concepts, somewhere out West. But I knew that that was not right for me either, that it was the West, and not the practice, that was attracting me.

I had hardened a bit, as naturally occurs, as I passed through my clinical training, wore my heart not quite so much on my sleeve. There had been, of course, Nepal and the events on the Tibetan border. But also, as an inevitable part of medicine, the non-logic of arbitrary death, disability, and disfigurement, seen at close quarters, does that to one.

I had taken care of too many four-year olds, vibrant and vigorous at three in the afternoon, and floppy and dying at seven in the evening from disseminated meningococcal disease, to leave myself as open as before. There is a dislocation of time for the young resident in the emergency room in those situations, a dislocation that never quite comes together again.

There you are, racing with your mind and body against the seconds and minutes on the clock, piecing together the story and sequence of events as related to you by the parents, while your own senses are gathering bits of information brought to you by your fingers and eyes and ears, working as fast as you can to draw the blood, perform the spinal tap without missing the tiny space of the canal or causing bleeding into it, getting the antibiotics started intravenously without tearing the lacy delicate vessels, difficult to thread into with the child already in shock. Time moving for you at ultra-high speed, while next to you stand the parents, stopped in time, their eyes wide and unmoving as their inner vision attempts to comprehend what they fear is happening to their child. Shuttled out into the waiting area, is it better for them to be spared the intimacy with frightful mechanical processes, or is it worse for them, forced to stand, or sit, or pace, in a cocoon of stopped-time, waiting for whatever word will come? For you there are endless combinations of possibilities, questions, explanations—what bug, what treatment, what shades of efforts and outcomes? For them there are only two things worth knowing: "Is she dead or will she live? Will she be all right, Doctor?"

Severe childhood trauma also provides the material for a lifetime's dreams, dreams that must be bulwarked against with a veneer of professional detachment. The possibilities are endless, and lie around every corner of thought: cars and trucks, bicycles, fireworks, falls from walls and trees, the pistol in the bedside drawer, sharp tools and dull weights, sticks and rock chips into eyes, ice and fire. And always the unexpected, the six-year old with a hand mangled in an old-fashioned clothes wringer discovered in the basement, bones and tendons and vessels and nerves squashed flat together.

Anger can be a defense for you against the consequences of the carelessness or stupidity of parents, but how can one remain angry at the young exhausted mother, herself a victim of earlier child abuse, who brought in her infant son with a broken arm and said to me, "I don't know why I do it, Doctor, but when he starts to cry and yell I just lose it and hang him up in the closet. I don't do it with his sister, just with him."

Not all the heart-hardening experiences come in acute packages of trauma or infection, not by any means all. There were the many severely neglected kids, like the twins we called the "Wolf Brothers," a pair about three years old who had no speech except what they recognized in the grunts and growls between themselves, and who crouched together all day in a single hospital crib and banged their heads against the rails.

One has to learn to say nothing while saying something to the many parents who wanted an explanation, any explanation, for why their child had been singled out for some horrible and agonizing fate, fast or slow, dramatic or insidious, invisible or impossible for the passerby to look at.

And then there were those with self-inflicted wounds. The winos and junkies in the adult emergency room with big livers and ulcerated needle-stick sores. The many young adults scraped off the road, who had learned the hard way about riding a motorcycle without a helmet, and that leather is not impervious to blacktop and gravel.

Yet there were many wonderful things as well, and I came to learn that it was those that truly formed one's shield, more powerful than the hardening of one's sensibilities against life's anguish and terrors.

All those kids who walked out of the hospital under their own power, when I didn't think they ever would.

All the courage of children, and of parents. And the courage of nurses who hung in there, year after year, on the children's leukemia ward.

All the people who said, "Thank you, Doctor," and meant it, and made you feel smarter than you knew you really were, and even once in a while sent a silly Hallmark card to you at the hospital.

And some of the senior doctors who knew so much, and applied it so easily, that you had to believe there was some trick to it, and could you ever learn it? Like the aging neurologist who examined small children by getting down on all fours on the floor and playing with them, often picking up subtle diagnostic clues that would be missed by the standard maneuvers. Or the fancy private practice clinician who would send patients to the hospital for work-up, and would say to the house staff, "You know, I think she might have (here insert some very rare and bizarre syndrome), what do you think about that?" and almost always be right. His name was Dr. Frankenberg, and we used to call his patients "franks and burgers." A call would come up from the Admitting Resident to the resident on the ward. "Oh, another frank-and-burger's coming in—get out the textbooks, but hold the mustard."

The Admitting Residents, who were senior residents on rotation, were identified by their juniors as either "Ironman" (the women as well) or "Sieve." It was up to "the Admitting" to decide which patients would be brought into the wards from the emergency room, and to schedule admissions from the private physicians who had privileges at the hospital. The private patient had to be admitted, unless the AR could talk the private physician out of it. As for the ER patients, it was up to the AR to make the final decision concerning the residents' views on whether a given patient was sick enough to be admitted to hospital. When beds were tight, or when the hour was late, and you were covering the wards and were "first up" for the next admission, you hoped that you had Ironman down there, and not Sieve.

So there was a lot going on for me in those years, and I worked hard at it, but at the same time I was floating through it, restless, waiting. I knew I had to get back "out there" somewhere, and that it would come, and that I had better be ready when it did.

And come it did indeed, like many things in my life, sort of out of the blue, and I never knew (and I have made it a practice never to ask too closely about these things) where it originated from, who talked to whom about what.

I got a phone call in the early summer of 1969. Would I come over to the State Department and talk with someone about something going on in Central West Africa?

The offices of the Director of the United States Agency for International Development's Office for Central West Africa were small and somewhat shabby, in a far corner of the main State Department building, in keeping with the general government principle that the longer the title, the less important and less impressive the digs. The Director himself was an easy-going sort, who seemed to know his stuff, but who readily admitted he knew nothing about mine.

"Here's the picture, Dr. Joseph. We have a request in for assistance from the Republic of Cameroon that looks interesting, but we don't think we have the capability to evaluate it. It seems that the World Health Organization, along with the Cameroon Government and assistance from the Canadians and the French, is starting a new medical school, which would be the only one in the country. The idea is to focus on producing doctors attuned to the real needs, and the realistic resources, that would be appropriate to an impoverished African rural society. What we don't want to get into down there is supporting another 'Disease Palace' that tries to put a stripped-down Massachusetts General in the middle of Africa. We thought that you, with your overseas time, and your recent Neighborhood Health Center experience, might be able to give us some realistic appraisal of the project. I also understand that you speak some French. We would ask you to go over for a week or two, and, while you are there, drop by some of the other countries in the region as well, and see what you think. We don't have any health programs going on, we don't have any health or medical staff on the ground, and I think it is a sector we ought to have some presence in out there."

The situation reminded me a bit of my recruiting visit to the Peace Corps. Just as I had been fundamentally ignorant about Nepal when the subject came up, in analogous fashion my only knowledge of Cameroon was limited to a dim memory of a few postage stamps in my father's own childhood collection. I thought it had been a French colony at the time, somewhere in South East Asia. Actually, "The Cameroons" had initially been a German possession on the West African coast, and after the First World War had been divided into British and French colonies. I was a little out of date, especially as the two halves had united at the time of independence around 1960. I had never thought much about Africa as a place I might want to work, except for the highlands in the mountain-spined countries of East Africa, the great plains teeming with game. My mental image, such as it was, of West Africa was of jungly closed-in sort of stuff, with pygmies peering around the roots of gigantic trees.

But a paid-for couple of weeks of medical tourism, and what sounded like an interesting intellectual problem, seemed an attractive prospect, and sure beat the same two weeks that would otherwise have been spent scheming as to how to screw a rival government agency out of a larger share of next year's Federal budget.

A week or so later, I flew from Washington to Paris. I walked around the world's most beautiful city for a day, trying to bring back my inadequately-spoken French, which had acquired a distressing tendency to come out half-Nepali, and then boarded the French UAL flight from Paris to Yaoundé, Cameroon. Yaoundé, now there's a name. Any place with more than twice as many vowels than consonants has got to have something going for it.

When you fly across the blue Mediterranean at mid-day, and then pass far above the gray-brown river of the Sahara for what seems like hours, and then gradually see the landscape below get greener and greener and the trees bigger and bigger, you feel that you have crossed all your known frontiers, and that you have arrived at someplace new and inexpressibly mysterious.

Yaoundé (how it rolls off the tongue in three and a half long syllables: *Ya/oww-oon-dey*) sits in a green bowl at more than two thousand feet above sea level, surrounded by the low silhouettes of green-forested and gray rock-ribbed mountains of rounded yet fantastic shapes. The fever-ridden coast is more than a hundred miles away, and Yaoundé lifts from the surrounding jungle, small farms, and cocoa plantations. Take the setting of some Lost World in the highland jungle of Brazil, squash it down a bit in scale and grandeur, set it down in West Africa, coloring everything a vivid green, and you have Yaoundé.

Despite the late afternoon hour, it was hot and muggy on the airport tarmac, and the sun possessed a fierce intensity I had not previously experienced, even high in the mountains. I was greeted by a junior officer from the Embassy, and hustled into a Land Rover somewhat the worse for wear (both me, from my long journey, and the Land Rover, from its own history). I was taken up to the Sheraton Hotel Mont Febe Palace, high on the tallest mountain overlooking the sprawling tin roofs of the small city, and, mercifully, left alone for a good night's sleep.

After breakfasting on dark rich coffee and fresh croissants at poolside (say, this wasn't so primitive after all!), I was picked up by Land Rover and uniformed driver and taken to the Embassy. The African driver, who was as big as a small refrigerator, and all dark glossy skin and white gleaming teeth, used the ten-minute drive to tell me all about how wonderful this city was, but how it was even more wonderful out in the home country of his tribe (Bamileke). I learned that his name was Jean-Chrétien, that he spoke French, English (a little), Bamileke, and Ewondo, had two wives and five children, and would be at my disposal while I was in Cameroon. I sat up front with him so that we could talk. In addition to this being instructive, it took my mind off the hair-raising, though skillful, manner of his driving, and the unfathomable and terrifying traffic patterns of Yaoundé.

All the American Embassies in small and seldom-considered countries in the 1960s looked pretty much alike. Gray concrete or white washed stucco, rectangular shape, the most elegant feature always the snappy Marine guard in dress blue pants, khaki blouse, and white top cover at the reception desk inside the front door. Two or three storeys: consular, public information functions, and minor administration on the ground floor, Ambassador's suite and his senior people on the second, and cable and cipher room, CIA, and military attaché up top. If it was only two storeys, the security and classified functions were squeezed in at the back.

"AmEmb/Yaoundé" was cut right out of the pattern. I was politely received by the Deputy Chief of Mission, who politely replied in polite terms to my polite pleasantries, and then was shuffled off to see the AID Mission Director, in a small corner building several blocks away.

There, not much was going on. The Mission Director, Hank Grady, was a youngish man, a U.S. Coast Guard Academy graduate and former officer, whose family descended from old-time fishermen in Marblehead, Massachusetts. I wasn't sure how that led to Central Africa. The rest of the staff consisted of John Montgomery, a jolly fellow who was serving out his time, and a slightly wacky but pleasant spinsterish secretary whom everyone seemed to refer to as "Our Nell."

All in all, it was not an overwhelming impression, but Grady was friendly enough, if slightly suspicious of what was the real message in Washington sending out this consultant to stick his nose in local programming decisions. I had the impression that Hank was concerned that this medical stuff might add significant complexities to his office routine, but still had something of an open mind, as it could potentially turn out to be a somewhat high-profile activity in a low-profile place, and move him up to a juicy plum for a next assignment, say, even, to Afghanistan.

We agreed that, after some initial briefing from Hank and John regarding the lay of the land and its context, and a very short "familiarization" tour to get an idea of some of the country surrounding Yaoundé, that I would spend several days with the Cameroonians and expatriates already involved in the medical school project, and then make brief visits to two of the other countries in the region, Central African Republic, and Chad (about neither of which I had any substantive knowledge). Then I would debrief with the AID office and the Embassy, and be on my way to deliver a report in Washington.

As I learned from Hank and John, Cameroon, sitting right in the hinge where the north-running coast of Africa makes a sharp ninety degree turn to the west, was primarily a rural country of several million inhabitants (no one was sure quite how many), and over a hundred and twenty tribal groups speaking almost as many separate languages and dialects. There were swamps and beaches on the coast, jungle in the middle, sometimes mountainous, and then tree- and grass- savanna sloping off to dry Sahel in the north. The Portugese seafaring explorers had originally named the area *Camaroes,* for the quantity and quality of the shrimp to be found off-shore. When the Germans ceded to the French and English after World War One, the two colonies developed along quite different lines and, of course, with different colonial languages, civil services, legal and educational systems, and currencies. As independence neared, West Cameroon, alongside the English-speaking Nigerian border, and East Cameroun, surrounded by other Francophone territories, decided in a plebiscite and a number of short but bloody border clashes, to form one nation. In addition to the divisions between Anglophones and Francophones, there were major differences between the Muslim tribes of the dry north, and the Christian and animist tribes of the forested south. In the short decade since independence, given that both the capitol, Yaoundé, and the major port city, Douala, were both francophone, the French culture and influence easily outstripped the British, and the young country fitted, for all intents and purposes, tightly into the French bloc of former West and Central African dependencies. There were residual animosities and tensions, but by and large the country was moving slowly forward in economic and other development terms.

All that Hank could tell me about the proposed medical school, aside from what I had learned in Washington, was that it was to be in Yaoundé, and was to be a part of the fledgling University, which had been developed along the French university model. However, it was the intention that the medical school itself, and the medium of instruction, was to function in both French and English. John had made an appointment for that very afternoon for me to meet with the Dean of the nascent school, Dr. Londe Korosso, who, evidently, was an Anglophone.

With Jean-Chrétien at the wheel of the Land Rover, and without running over any stray chickens or small children, I arrived at the temporary home of the "C.U.S.S" (*Centre Universitaire des Sciences de Santé* "U.C.H.S", *University Center for the Health Sciences).* The CUSS ("Kuus", as everybody, of whatever linguistic persuasion, called it) was housed in a three-sided collection of one-storey worn wooden barracks and storage sheds. Each of the adjoining offices, arranged motel-style around a hard-packed dusty yard, consisted of a cement floor, a desk and chair, a door, and, instead of glass windows, a cut-out wooden flap that could be propped open. There was an occasional bookcase, and one lecture room whose architectural style was identical to the offices, only larger and with more chairs. There was, intermittently, electricity, but the shade offered by the barracks was itself a welcome relief from the overpowering sun or the torrential rain, which alternated according to no discernable pattern.

And in this most unprepossessing place, I met a most extraordinary cast of characters, diverse in the extreme, and all powered, to various extents, by the same dream. Some of them were to become among my dearest friends.

Professor Londe Korosso, a West Cameroonian (and therefore Anglophone) academic internist, was deceptive, tyrannical, brilliant, and unscrupulous—just exactly the qualities one needed in the founding dean of a venture in as complex a set of circumstances as the CUSS. How he was able to push onwards the innovative and unconventional interests of this unlikely infant within the academic bureaucracy of an imitation-French university, I will never fathom, but always admire. Londe, as everyone called him, was a man never to take lightly, or at face value, or, even, at his word.

The World Health Organization team of resident advisors included an Israeli laboratory scientist as Chief of Party, an Egyptian pathologist, a French physiologist and expert in medical education theory, a Croatian nurse-administrator, and an Alsatian nurse-midwife.

Representing the Canadians were an anglophone male Public Health Physician who had grown up in a medical missionary family in Angola, and a francophone female nutritionist from Quebec. One can always rely on the Canadians for exquisite balance.

The French were represented by a Mutt-and-Jeff pair of young, well-trained, physicians. One, short, round, jolly and from Paris, was an internist. The other, tall, lean, and sardonic, was, of course, a general surgeon from Marseilles. Not by accident, and illustrating the intricate logic of French organizational planning, the wife of the internist was a dermatologist, and the wife of the surgeon was a clinical laboratory specialist who was especially expert in venereal diseases. Both were available for occasional drafts in teaching and consultation, though neither woman was officially part of the faculty.

The senior Cameroonian faculty consisted of a highly respected anglophone surgeon, who had taught previously at the medical school in Ibadan, Nigeria (the most esteemed medical school in West Africa), and who had performed exceptional medical service during the Biafran War. Now Vincent Ngoro, something of a national hero, had come home to serve his country. A young obstetrician-gynecologist, trained in the UK, had been recruited from his previous post as District Health Officer in the highlands of West Cameroon. There were rumors that a French-trained pediatrician would soon be arriving. And finally, there were four or five junior physicians, who were to act as teaching and clinical assistants.

The flight from Yaoundé to Bangui, the capitol of the Central African Republic, took somewhat more than two hours, over jungle that gradually gave way to dry and boulder-speckled plains. Bangui, formerly rather optimistically labeled the "Pearl of Central Africa," lay alongside a corridor of greenery formed by the Ubangui River. It was a former French Colonial town, with few buildings higher than a single storey, and much use made of shaded awnings and colonnades.

The CAR lay in the iron grip of a former French Army sergeant, Jean-Bedel Bokassa, who had seized power a few years earlier and now proclaimed himself "Emperor Bokassa." There were rumors of cannibalism in the "Palace", and on my first morning in town I heard a radio commercial from a local tailor who touted the wisdom of having one's prison clothes made to order *before* one was arrested. It was, to say the least, a spooky place, a house of mirrors overseen by a very sinister and very mad hatter, and my few days in Bangui were the first occasion (but not the last) when I, as a suspicious visitor, was followed in the streets by large dark men in even darker sunglasses. The government seemed to barely function, because of an equal admixture of indolence and terror. And yet there was a haunting beauty to the place: the dusty streets and the shaded stucco colonnades, the birds calling in the river trees, the endless forest and plain outside the town, the local Lebanese and Greek small shop-keepers, the women swathed in colorful cotton *panyas* (many of them with overprints extolling the virtues of the Emperor), wide-eyed babies stuck into a fold of cloth on their mother's backs, looking out at the world after it had gone by. There was an infinity of possibilities for needed health service projects, but I doubted the feasibility of doing any of them successfully, and left Bangui with only a twinge of regret.

I transited briefly back through Yaoundé, and then flew north to Chad, or as the French preferred to call it, Tchad. And there, in the capitol of Fort Lamy, a spell fell upon me, and my heart, or at least a great part of it, was lost to Africa.

"*Le Tchad*" (trust the French to coin an interplanetary name!) lay beyond any boundaries that one could even imagine. In the south were the great savannahs and marshes around Fort Archimbault. To the north, Sahel gradually gave way to the endless river of sand that was the true Sahara. Fort Lamy itself lay astride the magical Chari River, a dusty town awash in bright yellow light, white-robed and turbaned figures scurrying from one patch of shade to another. Old motorcars, kepi'd Legionnaires (there was a war going on in the north), fat old *colons* in white shorts and long white knee socks buttering radishes in the shabby hotel dining room, even a few side-glancing camels and magnificent Arabian horses in the streets and markets. Dry heat, so dry it sucked the spittle and sweat and moisture out of you, so that your body became desiccated enough to float upwards on your wildest dreams. The Last Outpost. The first step to a farther shore.

Though my major assignment was to assess the CUSS in Cameroon, it was in Chad that I first knew I must come to live and work in Africa.

Watel Bondo, the Director General of Health Services, was as black as he was tall and slender, with fingers so long that they were made for a surgeon's hands, and a reserved, almost regal, manner. He was one of only two Chadian doctors in the country, the rest being French military or *coopérant* physicians or Western missionaries. As I came to know later, he was an extremely competent surgeon, and worked extraordinarily long hours, operating in the mornings, and running the health services (such as they were) in the afternoons and evenings. Our meetings in his sparsely furnished Ministry office were formal, yet with an underlying ease and informality. To my surprise, on my last night in Chad, he invited me to have tea at his home. His wife was a delicately beautiful Frenchwoman with reddish-blond hair and a gracious manner. We talked until late into the evening on the verandah of their modest house, citronella candles keeping the mosquitoes at bay, and moths and bats flitting through the light. Seldom have I been as aware of what the New Africa could become. I was captured by the Bondos' mysterious elegance, the surrounding limitless darkness, the sense of a world so old and so new all mixed together, and, once again, that powerful attraction within me to the concatenation of medicine and adventure.

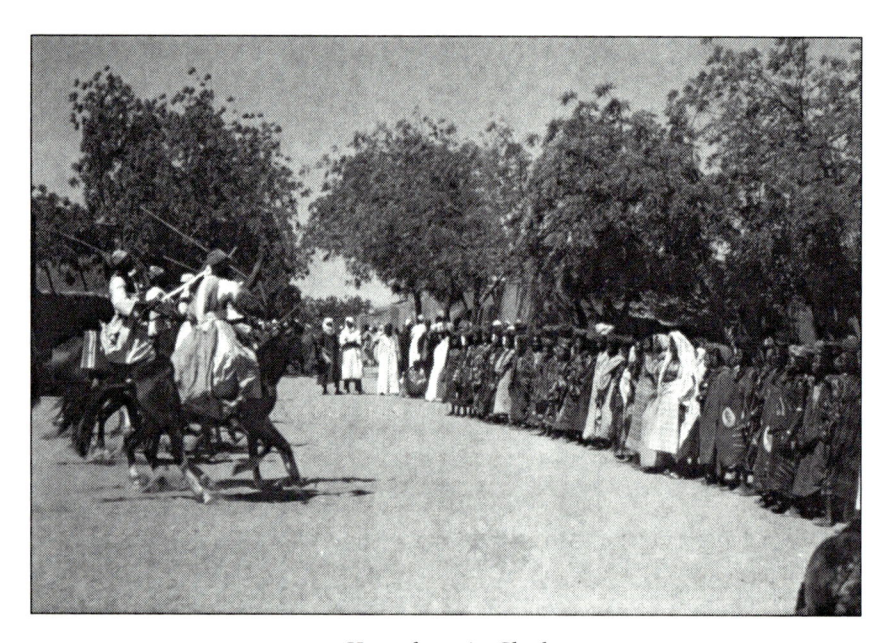

Horse fantasia: Chad

The U.S. embassy in Fort Lamy was a tiny place, but rather cheerful and relatively informal. It was awaiting the arrival of a new Ambassador, and the Deputy Chief of Mission in place, Jake Raines, was a rogue at heart. A softening form on a tall frame, in his mid-forties, he had bounced around the backwater posts of Africa for a decade, had seen it all and, while serious about his diplomacy, was not going to let anything over-ride his cynical sense of reality. Jake had risen about as high as he was likely to go, and I had the sense that that was all right with him. He may well have been a spook, and a good one at that. Jake was easy to get on with, told the most amazing African stories over a Scotch or two, and on my second evening in Fort Lamy said that he had two things to show me that would give me the whole picture.

Well before sunset we drove out of town along the road south to Fort Archimbault. Within five miles of Fort Lamy's outskirts, before the pavement gave out, we came upon a Land Rover parked on the verge alongside the road, thin forest on either side.

The roof on the driver's side of the Rover was crushed flat down, as if by a giant's foot, down to the level of the dashboard and front seat. Black stains and gristle residue could be seen beneath it. The left door lay under the chassis, and the right door hung open.

Gesturing with his hands, Jake explained: "Two French guys come down the road three days ago, about this time of day. They see a troop of elephants coming out of the forest on the left, and brake to let them pass. You can hear elephants coming a half-mile away, tearing off branches, knocking over trees and brush. There is no other sound like it. The troop crosses, and then these dumb bastards forget that an elephant troop most always leaves a rear-guard, usually an old bull, trailing along behind the cows and calves. So then they get the Rover into gear, move forward, and the old bull comes out of the woods, sees this elephant-gray box between him and his family, and just stomps the shit out of the Land Rover. The guy in the shotgun seat gets out and runs like hell back into town. The other guy wasn't so lucky."

Jake reversed the embassy Rover, and we drove back into Fort Lamy just as the darkness came on. He turned onto the main paved road (actually, the only paved road) leading north. For a short distance, as the center of town's mud-brick buildings fell away behind us, it was a wide boulevard, with a median strip holding flickering neon lamps. It was the road to the Presidential Palace. Halfway along there was a glittering fountain in the French Classical style. A fountain in the desert, lit by red and blue and white lights, which people stood around and watched, amazed at the miracle. But there was a further miracle still, a real one. In the grass along the median strip, under the lights, the young students of Tchad lay in the evening, reading their books, books that they might otherwise only be able to read at night by candle or lantern.

"There you have it," said Jake, and, oh, how I wanted to come back to Fort Lamy.

Back in Yaoundé, I spent a few more days going over details of the program with the CUSS faculty, talked with some students, visited some health centers and the *Hôpital Central,* got to know the nice young Peace Corps doc (who seemed an awful lot like me five years earlier), debriefed at the AID mission, and then flew home.

I wrote up a report on my trip, and made an appointment to deliver it along with an oral debriefing, and went over to the State Department building with a lot on my mind.

The Director leaned back and, puffing on a smelly pipe, listened to what I had to say.

"I think that the C.A.R is so nutty that there is little opportunity to do something constructive in the health field, and I didn't get to see Gabon or Equatorial Guinea (the other countries in AID's Central West Africa region), but I believe there is a real possibility for something very exciting and innovative in the CUSS in Cameroon, especially since Dr. Korosso is willing to take in some 'regional' students from Chad, and also the Ministry in Chad seems interested in a program to upgrade rural health centers. You'll see the detail in my written report, but I have a proposal to make to you."

The Director puffed on his pipe, and waited silently for what came next.

"If you get into this, you need somebody in the field to work it. So, why don't you send me over on a two- or three-year tour, let me work on health projects in the region, with particular emphasis on the CUSS, where Dr. Korosso says he'll give me a clinical teaching appointment if the U.S. joins the project."

The Director said nothing, just leaned a little further back, puffed a little more gently, and gave a half-smile. I realized then that I had been snookered, had walked straight into the snare that had been set for me. But,

I reasoned, the joke was really on him, because I was a more than willing captive.

So we worked out the details, and, just before the turn of the year, my wife and two small daughters and I boarded the plane for Paris and then Yaoundé. Following shortly behind us, by air, was one full-sized Collie (the Africans came to call him "Lion Dog"), and, by sea, one Volkswagen Camper Bus, which would take us where we wanted to go on those endless red dirt and mud roads of Central Africa.

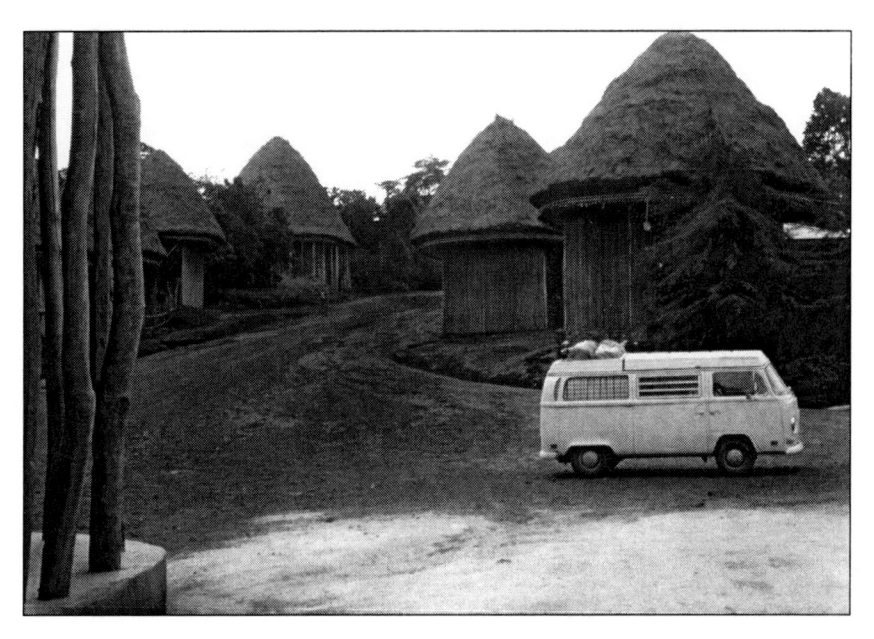

Camper bus in Bamileke village

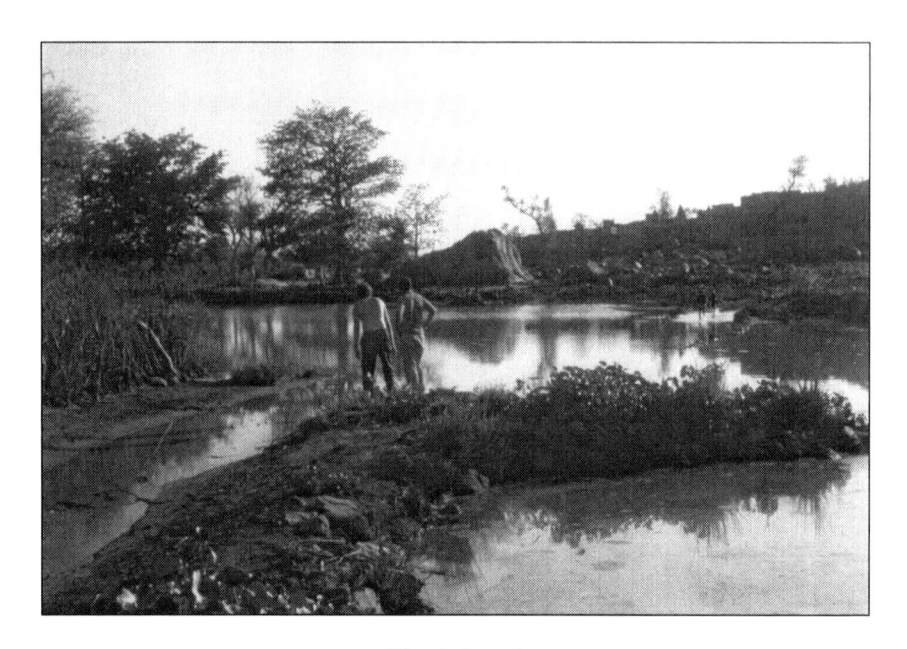

Flooded road

8

Yaoundé in 1970 sprawled among and between its green hills, climbing up to Mont Febe on the western edge of town, and fading off, as sprays and droplets from a splash of muddy water, along the red clay roads that led to who-knows-where. Stucco and cement at the center, mud-brick and tin roofs, and then mud and wattle as the roads led off and penetrated the surrounding forest.

In multi-layered Yaoundé's shallow ravines and lowermost plateaus were the shantytowns and slums that can be found everywhere in Africa: dirt lanes, more like paths really, unlit and sewerless, trampled into mud for half the year. Impossibly crowded, airless, lost forever from all the sustaining communality of the rural village, and yet possessing all the misery and poverty of those same communal villages, doubled and redoubled again.

Tentacles to the outside world: a small airport beyond the edge of town; a smoky, rusty train station, tracks leading west to the coast a hundred miles or more, and north to the interior Sahel; a beaten-earth plaza where dilapidated buses waited, strewn about like dominoes, interspersed with crowds, and vendors, and the universal buzzing human excitement of travel—to anywhere.

Off to one side, a sprawling market, stalls and arcades of poles and covering fronds. A medieval market: cloth, knives, house wares, fruits, bush-meat (mostly bush rat and monkey) and freshly butchered domestic meat, clouds of flies, chatter, laughter, good-natured pushing crowds.

I learned to take my medical students to the market on Friday mornings. We would stand and watch and see who could make the best and most clinical diagnoses just by observing.

"See there, over against that tree, those shriveled legs from polio.

Or there, the ivory eyes of trachoma. Coming slowly through the crowd, a sightless man led by a boy, each holding one end of a stick—blindness caused by the parasitic worm that makes its home inside the eye."

There were swollen limbs from filariasis, the occasional leper with missing digits, on and on and on. There would be the prize of a French chocolate bar for the most enterprising student of the day. Look and learn to see.

The town center consisted of two- and sometimes even three-storied cement buildings painted in yellows and pinks and blazing white. There were Greek and Lebanese and French businesses and shops, very few owned by Africans. Around them was the construction and trucking and heavier trades, almost all French-managed. A few restaurants existed, and many more food stalls on the side streets. On those side streets there were bars with open fronts and jangly music blaring from radios, color everywhere.

Climbing up the hills from the town center were the embassies, the walled and gardened residences of the expatriates. On the opposite plateau were the whitewashed government buildings, the military camp and the Presidential Palace.

Between the sectors, and separating them by class and caste like twisting fingers were fringes of green bush and trees. For every month of the year, these were a riot of color: tropical reds and yellows and oranges and pinks and whites. Flame trees, jacaranda, bougainvillea and flowering vines of a thousand aspects abounded. And birds. And snakes and rustling things. And people walking. Tall, short, round, thin black people, dark, dark black with glistening eyes and shining teeth and musical voices, and gesticulating hands. Graceful black women in bright colors, often with large bundles on their heads and small babies on their backs. It was rare to see a *blanc,* a European, afoot on the roads. But then, the sun was fierce, and the rain frequent and torrential.

The newly-rising University of Yaoundé lay along the flank of one of the eastern hills, modern concrete architecture set among the greenery. But the CUSS, the medical school, was not there, not yet. It awaited a permanent home, and resided, for the moment, lower down, wood barracks in a dusty dirt square off a secondary street.

My daily life lay divided among four places. First, a stucco villa in the expatriate quarter, surrounded by a flower-vined wall, set among small green trees and a vegetable garden. Once the gate was closed behind you, you might have thought you were in San Diego. But by night, a ragged *gardien* sat watch beside the gate, bow and arrow or machete at his side, nodding sleepily over a glowing charcoal brazier.

Second, the characterless Agency for International Development office, down the street from the American Embassy. I tried to spend as little time as possible at either.

Third, the CUSS barracks themselves, where my tiny office was, where my friends were, and where my students were, at least for lectures.

And finally, on a low plateau near the town's center, the *Hôpital Central* where I had charge of two wards: the "Under-Fives" children's ward, and a separate ward for children with measles. There was also a small, crowded room over in the obstetrical wing, where the premies were housed. There wasn't much we could do for them except keep them clean and fed (the former assured by the nurses, the latter by taking them to their mothers). For these premature infants we had four (inoperative) hospital incubators, donated by the tidy Dutch. Since there was no reliable electricity, the incubators served mainly as egg crates for two or even three premies apiece. If one became infected, we moved that baby to the regular ward, so as not to contaminate the others. Many survived, many did not.

The red tile-roofed hospital was built in the traditional French Colonial style, two verandá'd floors around a central open space. Electric power to the wards was intermittent; water ran mostly during the day, and was cold. Doors and windows were unscreened and hygiene, to say the least, uncertain. Next to the main buildings of the hospital was the *Protection Maternelle et Infantile (PMI)*, a bustling urban maternal and child health clinic. Mothers sat in line on crude wooden benches and waited patiently, their children in their laps or at their breasts. The PMI was the gateway for admission to my ward. Because of the ubiquitousness of serious illness and the eternal pressure on hospital beds, you had to be an extremely sick child to get into my ward. I was busy enough with the ones who passed the bar, and knew little of what happened to the ones who didn't.

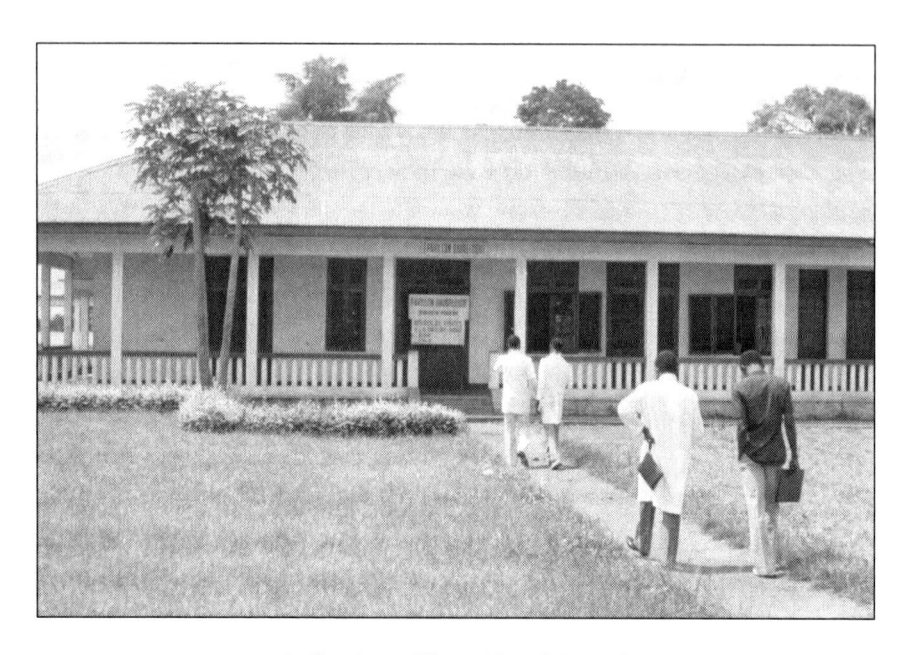

Pediatric pavillion: *Hôpital Central*

If I didn't have an early morning lecture, I spent the morning at the hospital, returning home at noon for lunch and at times a short siesta in the heat. Afternoons would be divided between the hospital, teaching at the CUSS barracks, or administrative chores (if they could not be shirked) at the AID office. At day's close, I generally performed a quick look-in at the wards. Most of my admissions from the PMI came in around ten or eleven in the morning, but occasionally a child more desperately ill than the other desperately ill children would arrive in the afternoon. It was rare to receive a night time admission, since the PMI was closed by late afternoon, and since there was no functioning public transport system in the town. There was a French-trained Cameroonian pediatrician, Chief of Service, who handled the older children's wards in the morning and his private clinic patients in the afternoon. We did not get on very well, but made a go of it, since each realized that the other was the only coverage he had. In the later years, I had medical students on the wards, but no interns or junior staff. The bulk of the work, as always, was done by the nurses. Most were women, most married with children of their own, and many, since the Central Hospital assignment was considered a plum, had significant professional or political connections. Almost without exception, they were serious, committed to their profession, and gave their best in the difficult conditions under which they worked.

The Under-Fives consisted of three large rooms, each holding fifteen or so beds. The metal cots were of one-size-fits-all, with stained mattresses and not enough sheets to go around. We had four or five cribs for some of the smallest infants, but most of the children lay in the larger beds. This was not such a bad arrangement, however, because the mothers slept in the beds with their children, and sometimes beneath the beds during the day. There was a nearby communal kitchen, where those mothers who were not breast-feeding their infants prepared their own and the patients' food.

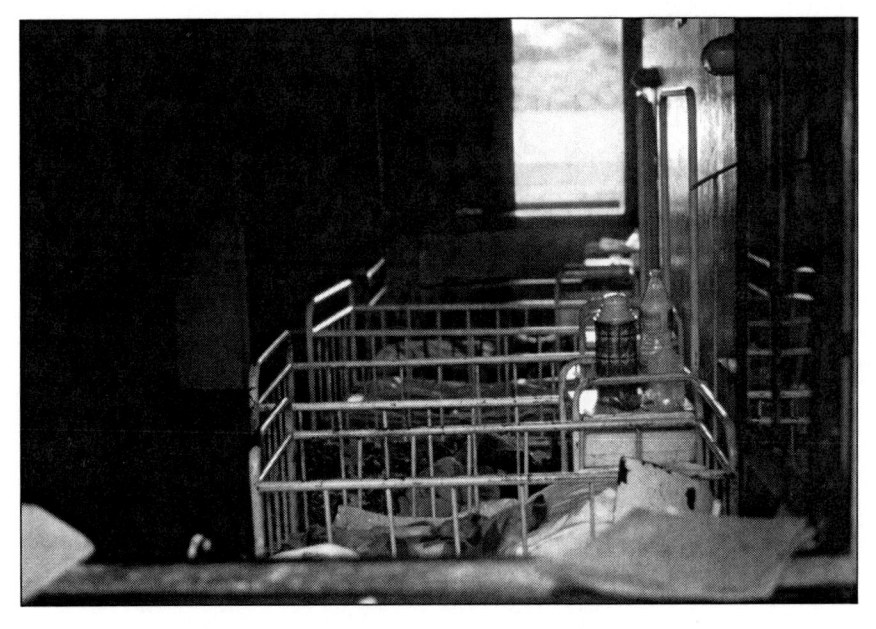

Under-fives ward: *Hôpital Central*

The walls were of frayed white-washed concrete, with one or at most two windows with swinging wooden shutters, which were invariably closed tightly at night, as was the glass-paned door that led out from the ward onto the veranda. The wards were always dim, if not dark, the electric light being insufficient by day, and usually powered off by night. In the center of each room was a wooden chair, and a rickety wooden table, which served the twin purposes of chart-writing and carrying out treatments, everything from physical examinations to inserting intravenous lines and doing spinal taps. Noise would have made it horrific, but in the gentle way that Africans have with their children, here was little screaming, and the usual background was one of mothers murmuring to the children as they stroked them or rocked them in their arms. Along one wall was a short tiled counter and sink. The counter could serve as a treatment area in a pinch, and the sink ran cold water intermittently, and dripped it constantly. At night, or when the shutters were closed during a rainstorm, I did my work by lantern, and made my rounds by flashlight. My spoken French rapidly became good enough that I could do everything I needed to do with the nurses. However, few of the mothers spoke French, and I depended on the nurses to serve as intermediaries for me in Ewondo, Bamileke, or a host of other tribal languages.

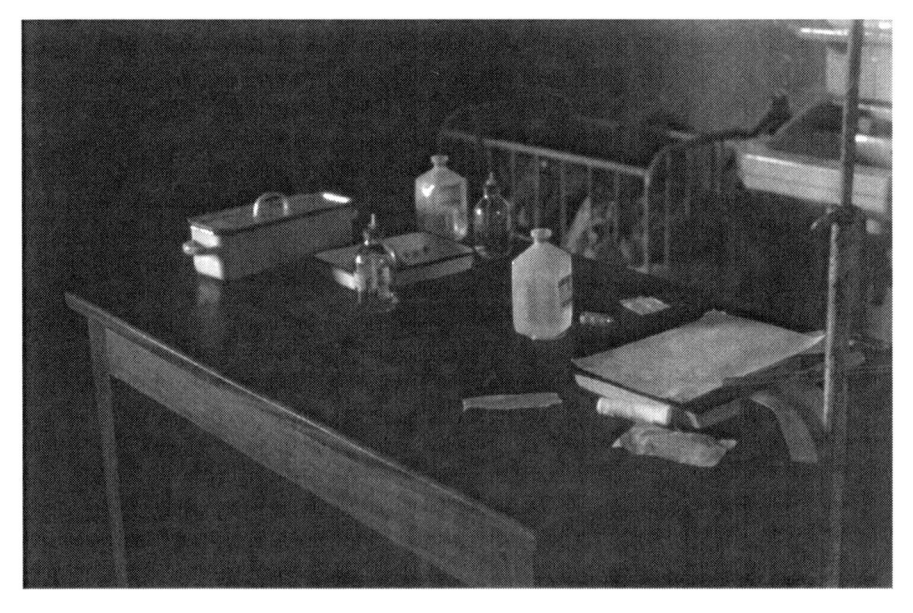

My work, examining and treatment table

Early in my work at *Hôpital Central*, I noted that many of the children I was treating had small fresh skin incisions, usually along the curve of their lower ribs over the liver. Then I realized that some of the children with such markings had not had, I could swear, those markings when I had examined them the day before. Bewildered, I asked the head nurse what was going on.

"Mon *Docteur*, you know that many of these mothers are not sure that we here can cure their baby."

And right they are, in all too many instances.

Madame Delphine, herself French-trained, and married to a senior official in the Ministry of Health, continued. "So to be sure that they have the best chance to get well, they carry the baby out from here at night, down to the Herbal Doctor, the how-you-say-Witch Doctor, down in the *quartier*. He gives them his treatments, and then the mother carries the baby back here, for us to treat in the daytime with our medicines. I think, perhaps, at times, this is not such a bad idea, no?"

I came to learn that my unknown colleagues' usual method was to make those small slits in the skin, and to blow into them insufflations of herb decoctions. I thought about it for a while, and then reasoned that my giving a sternly professional lecture in a language no one could understand, to mothers who didn't fully trust nor comprehend what I was doing anyway, would do no one, including myself, any good. Besides, I saw no serious inflammation nor other ill effects of the night-time procedure, and who knows, perhaps . . . ? Rumors persisted: that there was a foolproof native cure for jaundice, that "bone healers" could rub onto the skin a substance that would knit a broken bone in mere days. And darker rumors, as well, of illness "sent" to curse an enemy's child, or of exorcism to drive out the demon of an illness.

There were two fundamental differences in the characteristics of my patients in Yaoundé compared to those in Boston. Firstly, I had been taught to always try and reduce all signs and symptoms of a patient to a single unifying diagnosis, a single common pathway that would lead you to understand what the underlying disease process was. But these African children, almost without exception, had multiple distinct illnesses underlying what at last brought them to the hospital. Along with their pneumonia or diarrhea, they had chronic malaria, intestinal parasites, and, almost always, significant malnutrition. While the conditions were all interrelated, they also were all distinct.

Secondly, it was that mutually reinforcing combination of infection and malnutrition that brought them down and carried them off. Imagine, as you read this, not being able to feed your child well enough for health and growth, and then that child being exposed to a wide variety of serious infections, and then the inanition and fever of those infections compromising further his nutritional status, which makes him even more susceptible to the next infection, which...and round and round the fatal cycle spun.

Almost all mothers would breast-feed, adding small amounts of solid food but continuing to breast-feed for one or even two or more years. Themselves poorly nourished, their children faltered as the supply of mother's milk shrank, or as a new baby replaced the older one. Those few mothers who attempted bottle feeding without clean water, without refrigeration or a way to adequately clean the bottles, without the financial wherewithal to mix and sustain an adequately-concentrated formula—ended up with their infants much worse off than those who were breast-fed. Chronic and recurrent acute bouts of diarrhea sucked these children dry, of nutrients and adequate hydration.

There are two distinct types of early childhood malnutrition in Africa, and in Yaoundé I always had both on my crowded ward. Marasmus is the medical term for acute and profound starvation, usually occurring in the first year of life, though in times of war or famine (the "Biafran Babies") it can be seen at any age: stick-like extremities, swollen bellies, drum-tight skin over heads that seem outsized for the tiny wasted bodies. As I went about my work, the gazes of these children would silently follow me. They lay with an awful stillness: lethargic, hardly irritable enough to mewl with thin cries, their eyes dulled and expressions hopeless.

Kwashiorkor (from the Ga word meaning "the child displaced from the breast by the next-coming child") is aptly named. It most often occurs in children in the second or even third year of life, when for reason of privation or chronic illness, their malnutrition is dominated by an insufficiency of dietary protein. As they were brought in to the ward, from afar they could look almost robust, but their deceptive fullness was the result of edema fluid, sometimes so grotesque that their fingers and shins looked like plump sausages about to burst. Their hair was usually russet, if not overtly red, and on their cheeks and arms and legs there was a black scaly rash that looks like broken asphalt. These children also filled the ward, and their admission was usually prompted by acute and often overwhelming infection of one sort or another.

There are various gradations and intermediary states between marasmus and kwashiorkor, but a pattern common to them both is the child who is just balancing on the knife-edge of clinically severe malnutrition, and who then gets a bout of diarrhea, or pneumonia, or measles, or severe malaria. The child burns off calories from the fever, doesn't eat or drink well for a few days or a week, and tumbles off that knife-edge. Does the predisposing malnutrition "cause" the collapse? Does the infection "cause" the loss of a fragile equilibrium? It hardly matters, the result is the same.

I treated a constant stream of early childhood infections on my ward: meningitis, septic joints, mastoiditis, cerebral malaria, tetanus of the newborn, polio. But the underlying factors most frequent among my patients were common diarrhea or pneumonia (or both) on a base of marasmus or kwashiorkor. From the records that I kept, fully fifteen percent of all the children I admitted died on the ward, and over half of that number expired from malnutrition with associated diarrhea and/or pneumonia. Under the pressure of large numbers of children, all desperately ill, I learned to examine patients quickly, not pause to put too fine a point on what might or might not be there (in other words treat everyone for worms and chronic malaria if they were strong enough to handle it), and to go aggressively for the obvious, without waiting for laboratory confirmation. Since medical history-taking was inadequate, the mothers and I speaking a different language in more senses than one, I tried to hone my physical diagnostic skills to as sharp an edge as I could, to think and act decisively on the basis of what my eyes and hands could tell me, with a stethoscope thrown in for good measure. We did have a laboratory in the hospital, which gave me routine blood counts, malaria smears and bacterial microscopic identification and so forth, not much in the way of blood chemistries, and nothing reliable regarding bacterial cultures. X-ray was available, if I went and hunted down the films myself and didn't wait for a report to come back. If I was really in a hurry, I carried the child across the courtyard, and stood over the technician as the film was developed. The blood bank was passable, used mostly by the surgeons.

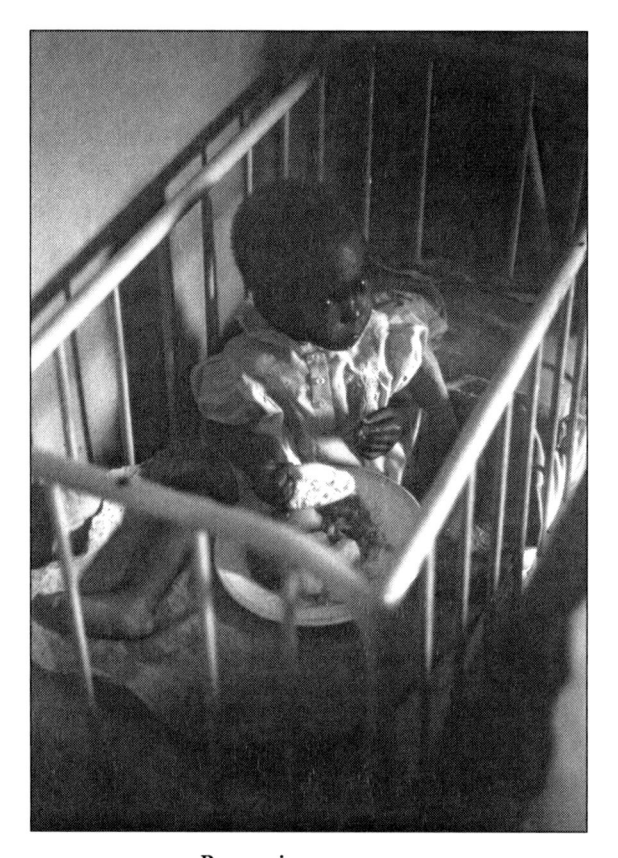

Recovering marasmus

Supplies and medicines were a major problem. Antibiotics would often run out toward the end of the month. The minor sterile supplies: needles, syringes, equipment for intravenous fluid administration and venous cut-downs, and lumbar punctures—all of which I used at a steady clip—were in poor condition and often lacking. I got in the habit of begging the used disposable needles from the American Embassy, sharpening them on a whetstone, and re-sterilizing them again and again. It was crude, but effective. I must admit that when things got tight, I was not above surreptitiously liberating a bottle or a vial of needed antibiotic from the embassy health room. I'm not sure anyone would have minded, but I didn't take the risk of asking. Besides, I figured that it was fair compensation for all the free medical care I provided to the American community. What we used to call that, back in Boston, was "Robin Hood Medicine," stealing from the rich to give to the poor.

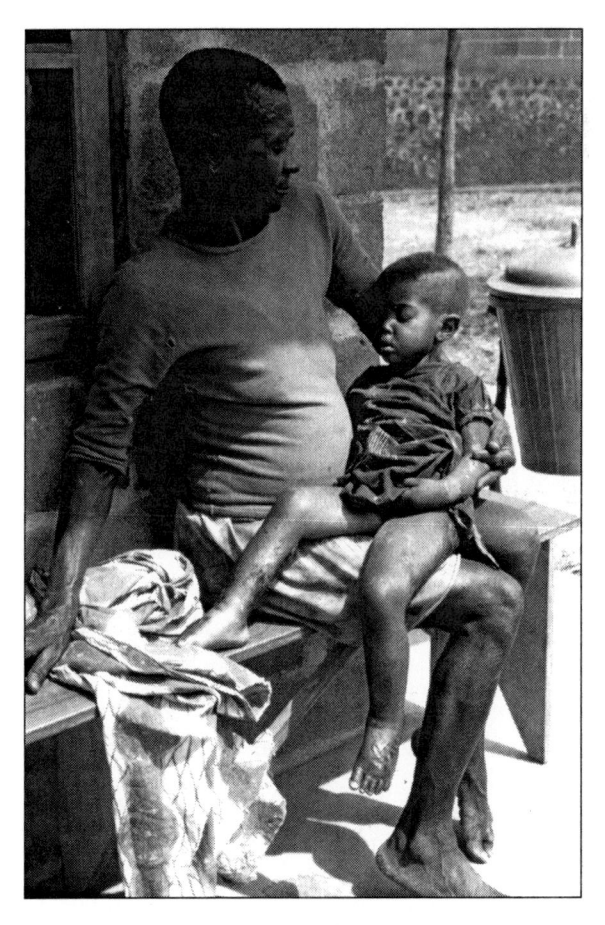

Kwashiorkor

Because of the difficulty of keeping IVs running in tiny and fragile veins under the ward circumstances, I did many more "cut-downs" than would have been thought proper back in Boston. The African nurses were incredibly dexterous at this procedure (which involves dissecting down through skin and subcutaneous tissue upon a more or less superficial vein, freeing it up, making a nick in it without cutting through it entirely, tying off the upstream end, and slipping a slim catheter up into the downstream end, secured with a suture), and I came away with some new tricks for speed and accuracy. I did spinal taps and aspirated joints by the barrel-load. The mothers would stand over my shoulder, but never say a word. I have often heard it said that mothers in poor countries are "stoic," that they grieve less for their children "because they are so used to losing them." In my experience, this is not true. And I have had plenty of experience of telling African mothers that their child is dead. Their grief is as deep and genuine, I believe, as that of any suburban matron.

So, pneumonias and diarrheas, antibiotics and intravenous fluids (I was at that time ignorant of the efficacy of sugar/salt oral fluid administration, which was just coming into use) and antibiotics. Try to get ahead and stay ahead on both counts.

Because so many of my patients were clinically malnourished, I thought that teaching the mothers to make a high-protein feed with locally-available ingredients would both improve the children's survival rate in-hospital, and give them a better chance to stay alive after they went home. The Canadians had sent over a clinical nutritionist as part of their team, and I asked Helene DuRose to start a demonstration kitchen on my ward. She met, I regret to say, strong opposition from the nurses: "It isn't done that way." "She is not a nurse, and doesn't belong here." "The mothers don't use those sorts of foods." We persevered, but without great success. Lest any readers feel unduly smug about "ignorance," they should think about the likelihood of changing the dietary patterns of themselves or their own families, even when disease prevention benefits are known.

Many of the diseases that filled my wards are easily preventable by prior immunization. Tetanus of the newborn requires but a single injection given to the mother late in pregnancy. Measles can be totally prevented by a single injection given in Africa at six months of age. Whooping cough and polio are averted by a series of immunizations in infancy. Diphtheria is very rare in African children, and this is thought to be due to early exposure to diphtheroid organisms as skin infections, a crude unwitting form of immunization. Smallpox was on the verge of eradication in West Africa in the early 1970s, and I never saw a case of smallpox on my urban children's ward, though I saw several very malnourished children who had severe reactions to the vaccination. A vaccine against meningococcal meningitis was just coming into use, but was not yet widely available in Yaoundé. These various immunizations were unlikely to be available to provide protection for the children of Yaoundé's slums, or to the children of the surrounding villages, and I treated the results.

For me, perhaps, the most frustrating disease was neonatal tetanus. Completely preventable, as stated above, by a single injection during pregnancy, or the use of a sterile razor blade to cut the umbilical cord at delivery, or the avoidance of rubbing mud, animal dung, or hearth ashes on the cord. Once the disease developed, usually toward the end of the first week of life, there was little I could do. I lacked adequate supplies of antitoxin. I administered antibiotics, but the germs that produced the deadly circulating toxin were usually long-gone by the time the disease was fully developed. The slightest disturbance of the infant—a breeze of air, a noise, a bright light, a mother's gentle handling, feeding—these would set off the agonizing spastic convulsions of arms, legs, trunk, neck, and face. I gave as much sedating barbiturate as I dared, placed the crib in a dark corner with a cloth over the top, and, with the mother, waited it out. Half of these neonates survived, half did not.

Polio was another heartbreaker. By the time they reached my ward, these children were long past the initial "minor illness" that precedes the paralytic stage. Most came late, well after a leg was flaccid and paralyzed. They would sit propped against a wall, the useless limb flopped out in front of them, eating their gruel from a metal pan; there was literally nothing I could do for them. A few came in with respiratory distress from chest wall paralysis, or comatose with brain stem involvement. I had no way to sustain long-term respiratory support for those patients. They either recovered or, most of them, died.

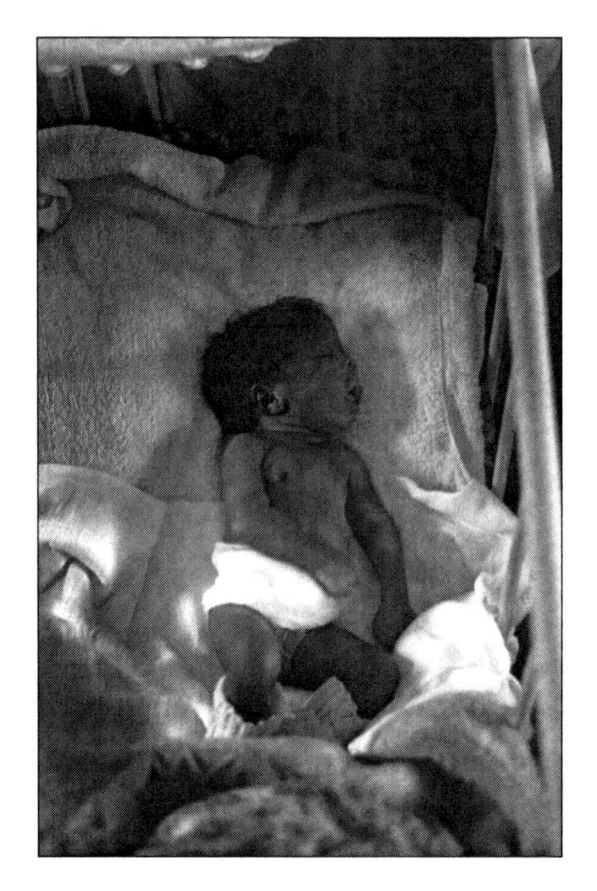

Tetanus Neonatorum

The measles ward was an isolated narrow hall at the other end of the hospital, down past the adult wards. There was a door, kept closed, at one end, and a window, usually also closed and with its panes painted over, at the other. The room was kept in semi-darkness, because of the painful sensitivity to bright light of many of the patients. In the room were 20 small beds, lined along each wall, with a narrow corridor between. The beds were always full, with at times two patients to a bed.

Measles in West African children is a far, far different disease than what I had known, before the advent of the vaccine, in America. It affected mostly children in the second half of the first year of life, or shortly thereafter, instead of being the school-age infection that I had experienced in America. African babies are not home alone. Constantly in a communal knot of women and children, carried on their mother's back, or set down with others alongside her as she pounds the grain or tends the fire along with the other village women, they mix with other babies, other children, and adults. In the early 1970s, before the widespread availability of immunization, huge outbreaks would sweep across local regions, usually on a two-yearly basis, and almost all susceptible children would become infected. Compounding the problem of measles itself was the timing—often just when malnutrition was becoming significant. During the period of a week or ten days when the child suffered the fever, dehydration, and diminished food intake associated with the measles, with or without complications of pneumonia, ear or eye infections, encephalitis, he or she was often precipitated into acute malnutrition, usually kwashiorkor. Because we received the sickest patients (those who were not sent home from the PMI to infect others), one in five of my measles children died during their disease.

That did not include the ones who went home deaf, blind, or brain-damaged, and did not include the children whom were discharged "recovered" from the measles, and whom I recognized two or three weeks later, returning this time to enter the Under-Fives ward, with fulminating kwashiorkor and some other associated deadly infection.

Pneumonia, diarrhea, malnutrition—these I could accept, in a sense, as the currency of poverty. But tetanus, polio, measles, and whooping cough—all completely preventable by immunization—each one of these that I treated, successfully or not, represented a downstream failure, something that could have been averted with tools we had and knew how to use. They made a mockery of the old saw: we did not apply an ounce of prevention, and we did not possess, by a long shot, the requisite pound of cure.

It was on a Sunday morning, and happened to be one of the final days of the month. I was standing in my Under-Fives ward, doing a quick rounds with Madame Delphine, the Head Nurse. As I remember it, we were in a far corner of the room, whispering so as not to set off another series of convulsions in the small baby with tetanus, who lay in a crib nearby covered with gauze to keep out light and breeze.

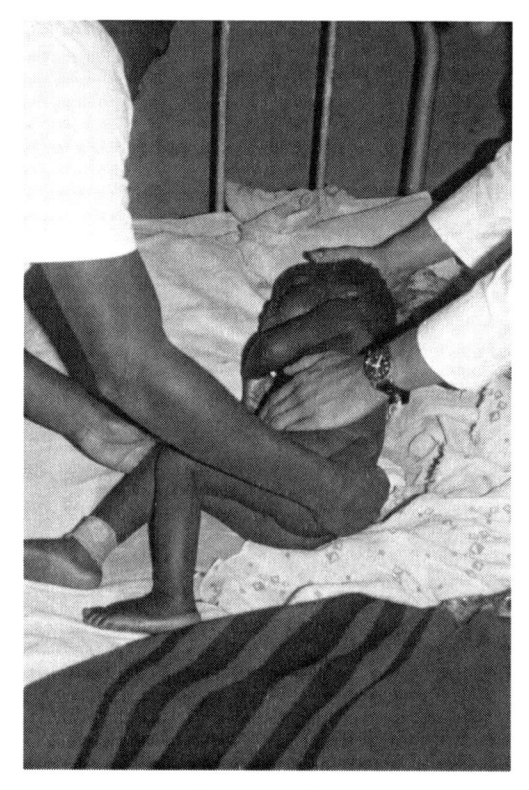

African measles

Through the ward doorway, backlighted by the sunshine, I saw a woman dressed in a green *panya*, carrying in her arms what appeared to be a loaf of bread, itself draped in a cloth.

But wait, that can't be a loaf of bread. There is an arm hanging from it. And that is a child's head, tipped sharply back, at one end.

Delphine was faster to react than I was. With one arm she swept clear a space on the counter which we used as an examining table. With the other arm she guided the woman toward the counter, and then gently took the child from the mother and laid it on the counter. Simultaneously, it seemed, she called to an assistant nurse, "Honoré, run and get an IV pole, an infusion set-up with Dextrose and water, a spinal puncture set, and a cut-down tray. Vite! Vite!"

As I began to rapidly examine the child, Delphine translated for me the responses of the Ewondo mother to my questions. I listened carefully, but kept my eyes and my hands on the child.

"*Docteur*, she has run all the way here from the *quartier* with the baby, who is three months old, and seemed well today until he had a convulsion about an hour ago, and he has been like that, like he is now, since. She could feel him shaking in her arms as she ran up the hill. No, he has had no cough or diarrhea, and no recent fevers. *Docteur*, she wants to know, can you give him some medicine?"

Speaking half to myself as I examined the child, and half to Delphine: "His neck is stiff as a board, and he won't let me flex it. He is unconscious, with his eyes rolled back. He clearly has a high fever. Heart okay, nothing in the lungs, ears and throat are clear, no sign of trauma, no obvious skin lesions. His belly is soft, with a somewhat enlarged liver and spleen—like most all the kids here he probably has chronic malaria, but that is not, I think, his problem now. This is not cerebral malaria, this is meningitis, maybe generalized sepsis as well, and we don't have much time to get on top of it."

As if in answer to my comments, the boy spasmed in a sudden convulsion, and then went completely rigid. His breathing was rapid and shallow, his pulse was thready.

Delphine was already splashing cool water over him in an attempt to rapidly lower the fever, even as I was rolling him on his side, cleaning his back with iodine, and pulling on a set of gloves as the assistant nurse opened the spinal puncture set.

Honoré held him on his side for me, slightly curled despite his rigidity, to flex open the vertebral spaces and make my task easier.

I slid the needle in, pulled out the stopper, and what spurted out under high pressure looked like pure pus. Even while I was doing the spinal tap, Delphine was prepping the side of the child's ankle for a venous cutdown, and she finished the procedure just moments after I had collected some spinal fluid in a tube, taken the spinal needle out, and rolled the child over onto his back. All this while the mother stood closely by, making not a sound.

"Okay, Delphine, keep working on the fever and hang up the D5W solution. There are some Tylenol suppositories in my bag in the corner. Break one in half and insert it." (I had stolen them from the Embassy Health Room the day before.) I did some quick mental calculations for dosages, jotted figures on a scrap of paper, and said, "Honoré, just as fast as you can, get these amounts of Ampicillin and Gantrisin pushed in quickly through the IV. I'll give you the on-going dosages later. And, yes, let's give him some IM Chloroquine, for malaria, just on general principles. And have the oxygen and an AMBU ready, and the emergency box handy, just in case. And . . . "

"*Docteur*," said Delphine quietly. "There is no Ampicillin. We ran out yesterday, and the hospital pharmacy will have no more until next week, nor have they any form of penicillin left for this month."

I reached in my pocket and threw several CFA thousand franc notes on the table. "Have someone run as fast as they can to one of the downtown pharmacies, and get what we need."

"*Docteur*," it is Sunday morning. The Pharmacie Centrale and all the others, they are closed."

"Dammit! Honore, leave that IV to me. Run over to the Medical ward, and see if Dr. Pierre is there. Get some Ampicillin from him. Tell him it is urgent."

We pushed in the Gantrisin and injected the Chloroquine, and then stood counting the seconds, waiting for the child to stop breathing. He had another convulsion.

Honoré reappeared, followed only a few steps behind by a puffing Vincent Ngoro. The surgeon caught his breath, and stammered, "Steve, I was standing talking with Pierre when your nurse came. I have no Ampicillin, and I think there is none in the hospital, but I did have some crystalline Penicillin G stashed in my office fridge, so here it is. Always save a little in reserve, that's what I learned in Biafra. Use all you want."

"Thanks, Vincent, I'll replace it from the downtown pharmacy tomorrow. I owe you one."

We ran in the IV Penicillin as fast as we could. I made a few notes, wrote a few orders for the next 24 hours' care, and ran off to the side room to run a few lab tests. The spinal fluid was grossly purulent, and when I did a Gram stain of the sediment, under the microscope, in addition to the innumerable white blood cells, it was full of classical "Gram-positive diplococci"— in other words meningitis with the common pneumococcal bacteria that were exquisitely sensitive to penicillin. A thick smear of the blood, of which Delphine had let some run out into a few tubes as she did the cut-down, revealed malaria parasites, but not too many. I sent a tube of the blood over to the bank for type and cross-match, should we need it later, and another tube to the bacteriology lab for culture, even though I had the answer, and the blood was not sterile as it was collected.

I went to tell Delphine the good news, that we had a treatable infection and the means to treat it, and found her standing at the child's side with the mother, talking to her softly, her arm around the woman's waist.

"Delphine, tell her that her baby is very sick, with an infection in his brain system, but that we have the right medicine for it, and we will do everything we can to save him, and hope that we can. She can stay here with him, and you and I will answer her questions. Tell her she did exactly the right thing to run here as fast as she could. Exactly the right thing, and that she should be proud to be such a fine mother."

The woman, who appeared to be about eighteen years old, would not look directly at either Delphine or myself; she kept her eyes lowered to the floor, but she slowly nodded her head when my words were translated into Ewondo. With her left hand she was stroking her baby's thigh.

"Madame Delphine," I said in my best and most formal French. "Surely and without question, you are God's gift to this place."

"Oh, Mon *Docteur*," she said shyly, as she poked an elbow into my ribs, which she had never done before. "We only do what work we can, is it not so?"

We stood and watched the child for a bit, hoping we could see the magic medicine do its work. The child remained comatose, but the fever did come down, and there were no more seizures.

I left the ward for an hour or two. I dropped by home, which was only fifteen minutes away, then came back to the hospital to thank Vincent again and tell him his penicillin might make all the difference. I stopped by to check on the measles ward, where things were as horrific as usual, and then I went back to the Under-Fives to see how things were going.

As I approached the veranda and the ward entrance, a woman in a green *panya* came out from the interior shadow of the ward. In her arms was what appeared to be a loaf of bread. But this time the burden was completely wrapped and covered.

As she stepped over the threshold, I could see the tears streaming down her face, but she made no sound that I could hear. She stumbled on the doorsill, and almost fell. But she didn't drop what she was carrying.

And so I worked in my vineyard, soiled though it was, sometimes in tragedy and occasionally in triumph. I thought often, and carefully, about my medical students. In all likelihood, they would have to prepare for a lifetime of service under the conditions in which I was now working. I would depart, sooner rather than later, and go back to a privileged environment. But the best of them, those who did not flee to France or Britain, who stayed to work to build their young country, could only look forward to changing the conditions such as those in the *Hôpital Central* bit by bit, if at all.

What was the most useful education and training I could offer them? How to balance the teaching so that it did not dangle before them unattainable standards, but at the same time did not look down on them? Was there any way for an outsider to feel his way through this dilemma? The best I could come up with, though I did not rest easy with it, was "focus on the practical, emphasize self-reliance and tenacity, and convey to them your pride and respect for what they aspire to."

The CUSS, in my view, was a magnificent concept, and as all such concepts are, it was riven by internal contradictions. In the midst of a society that could not feed nor protect its children, the idea was to train young physicians who were suited, and motivated, to staff the rural health centers and ramshackle hospitals, to have skills sophisticated enough that they could make a maximum of difference in those settings, but not so sophisticated that they would be ill-suited, educationally and psychologically, to remain there.

The major problem lay not so much with the students as with us, their teachers. We ourselves, whether European or African, were ill-trained for the task of producing rural primary care physicians for Africa, being formed as we were in the subspecialty and technologically dominated atmosphere of the modern tertiary hospital. We had our own ambivalence concerning what was needed, and what was adequate. All of us, including the Cameroonians, had been trained in the "Disease Palaces," the sub-specialty hospital environments of European and American medical schools. Despite what we saw as the impossibility, and even non-desirability, of "imposing" that model on a country with near-universal poverty, rudimentary infrastructure, and a total health care budget of less than two dollars per person per year, it was difficult for any of us to truly commit ourselves to a different course of action, however logical or necessary it might seem.

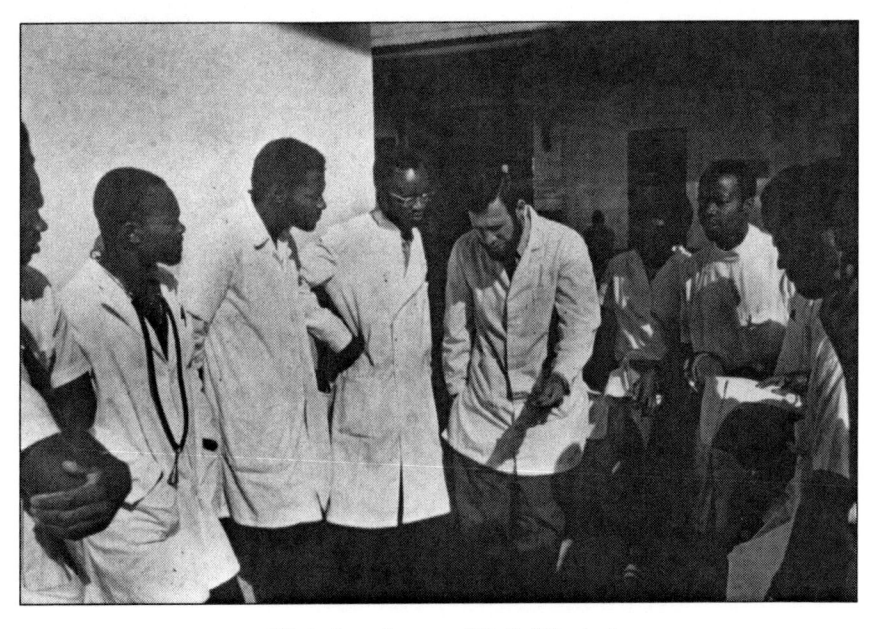

Clinical conference: *Hôpital Central*

At its most simplistic, the argument boiled down to "are we training *real doctors* or not?" On another level, the African faculty, who had the greatest stake in the issue, at times suspected more than a whiff of colonialism (neo- or otherwise) in the air. And beyond this there were the not-insignificant cultural and medical watersheds that often separated the expatriate partners. The Canadians, and myself as the lone American, usually stuck together and took the hardest line, somewhat self-righteously at times I fear, in support of focusing on outpatient primary care and rural health services. The French, often exhibiting a "pride of place" as the former colonial authority, were quite skeptical about these heretical ideas, and wanted to be sure that the proper focus was placed on hospital medicine and surgery. The World Health Organization fancied itself as the intellectual authority, *primum inter pares*, but provided mostly pre-clinical faculty, and therefore had less credibility with those of us whose feet were more firmly planted in the mud.

And the Cameroonians, pulled and pushed by these various factions, dependent on the external resources that flowed from (or might be with-held by) the expatriate groups, must have had legitimate questions as to whether they were, in fact, masters in their own house. Dr. Londe Korosso, the Dean, and a proud and ambitious man, had to navigate these treacherous currents and balance the competing interests. In the end he was able to please nobody, but he skillfully kept the team together, and the institution growing.

The Americans, as usual, had the most money to spend. As part of the program of assistance that I was shepherding through USAID, we were to finance and to provide the architect for the construction of "the New CUSS"—administrative space, teaching facilities, library and laboratories, and clinical facilities. But, and this was a big but, those clinical facilities were not going to be at the Central Hospital, but were rather to be outpatient clinics in the form of an urban health center. When, after having negotiated this proposal with Dr. Korosso, it was presented to the faculty, the Canadians were strongly supportive, the WHO was on the fence, and the French were dismissively critical. As for myself, I was only too conscious of the irony that pitted my conceptual position against the realities of my daily practice.

An American architectural firm was engaged to do the design, and fortunately was able to work with the French university authorities (the rector of the University of Yaoundé at the time being a noted Parisian academic) and with the diverse perspectives of the CUSS faculty, without too much crockery being broken. And in the end, the possibility of moving out of our dusty wooden barracks into what became a quite beautiful and reasonably functional "real" medical school, proved an irresistible magnet.

In those early years, to emphasize the primary care and rural health aspects of the program, the CUSS created two clinical teaching programs that every student had to rotate through. The first was an improved urban health center, a mile or so from the CUSS itself, which was to serve as a teaching focus until the new facility was built. A young Anglophone Cameroonian physician from the faculty, herself trained in pediatrics in the United States, supervised this program, which included sick and well child and maternal care, immunization clinics, and home visiting. The Canadians added public health and nutrition functions. The French internist and surgeon sniffed, and focused on their hospital teaching.

The second program was more ambitious, more difficult, and more controversial. We designated the "Bamenda Rural Health Project" in the District of the same name, where there was a quite good district hospital and a ring of rural health centers. What made this ambitious, difficult, and controversial was that the Bamenda District was almost two hundred miles away from Yaoundé, up in the high grasslands, and Anglophone environment, of West Cameroon. Distance, language, and a quite different medical/cultural tradition than that of the French-majority environment of the CUSS in Yaoundé all combined to present formidable obstacles.

The plan was that groups of fourth-year medical students (the CUSS curriculum was based on a six-year French university medical school model) would spend an eight-week block living and working in Bamenda District, at the rural health centers, the district hospital, and with the mobile immunization services. Even more heretical, each "team" would consist of not only medical students, but also students from the nursing school, working jointly to produce a research project of their choice, to be presented to the faculty at the end of the eight-week period.

The French sniffed even more loudly this time, judging this to be a waste of precious curriculum time. A young Belgian WHO physician volunteered to move himself and his wife (a nurse) and infant son up to Bamenda as full-time faculty for the program, and other WHO, Canadian,

American, and Cameroonian faculty all pledged to keep at least one additional faculty member up in Bamenda on rotation, a week or two at a time. Though the promise was sometimes most honored in the breach, it probably did more than anything else to keep the underlying concept of the CUSS from deteriorating into "just another medical school."

Going up to be with the students in Bamenda, for which my VW Camper Bus was the perfect vehicle, was great stimulation and a great joy. I drove through dense forest on red laterite roads, passing through thatched villages. Coming out of the forest on the edge of the grasslands, I was in the savanna, dotted with baobab trees and large rock outcroppings. Troops of baboons would bark from the road margins. Then, up on the grasslands themselves, the views across the rolling hills went on forever. Higher and cooler, the government stations and health centers were often built as stone cottages, surrounded by eucalyptus. On the edge of the grasslands, to the west, the land fell away steeply into dense tropical forest. And, I am slightly ashamed to say, there was a good old *British* feel to it all, including to the health services, that was just more easy and comfortable for an American than the constant effort of conforming to a French environment and medical culture.

The CUSS students were about one-third Anglophone and the balance Francophone. They were all supposed to be bilingual, but in Bamenda, for the first time, they had to work in an Anglophone medium and environment. The nursing students, from the school at the district hospital, were Anglophone. We mixed up the teams so that each had at least one Anglophone, and the students did remarkably well.

I can't say that all the students loved the Bamenda experience. Some would complain bitterly about being "in this isolated bush, where there is nothing to eat." But they did well, and learned how to work with the nurse-midwives of the rural health centers. The CUSS students coped as best they could with night time emergencies, often without electricity, running water, or adequate staff or supplies. They experienced first-hand the difficulties of immunizing children on a mobile basis, of getting mothers to return on a regular basis for preventive care and nutritional advice when their children looked healthy, and it was a long walk to, and a long wait at, the health center. They selected simple problems to research, such as the prevalence of this or that type of parasite in children attending the health center, and saw the projects through, wrote them up, and presented the results.

Most importantly, I think, they gained an idea of what the probable future held for them as young physicians. Some would have the desire or the connections to leave Cameroon immediately after graduation for specialty training in France or England. But most would serve, for at least a number of years, as physicians in the major rural health centers, or in the rural hospitals. Bamenda gave them a foundation on which to build.

What I tried to teach my students (and myself) on the wards of the *Hôpital Central* and in the Yaoundé marketplace was, of course, the irreplaceable substrate of a life in medicine. But, somehow, I think that also Bamenda was an equal part.

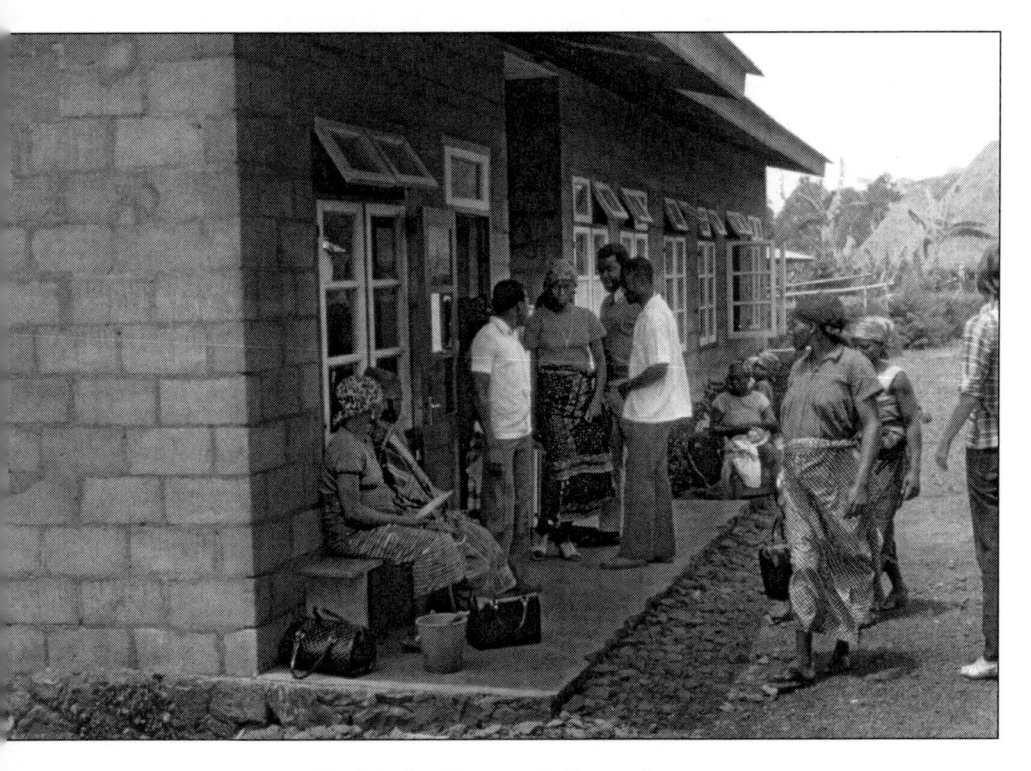

Teaching health center in Bamenda

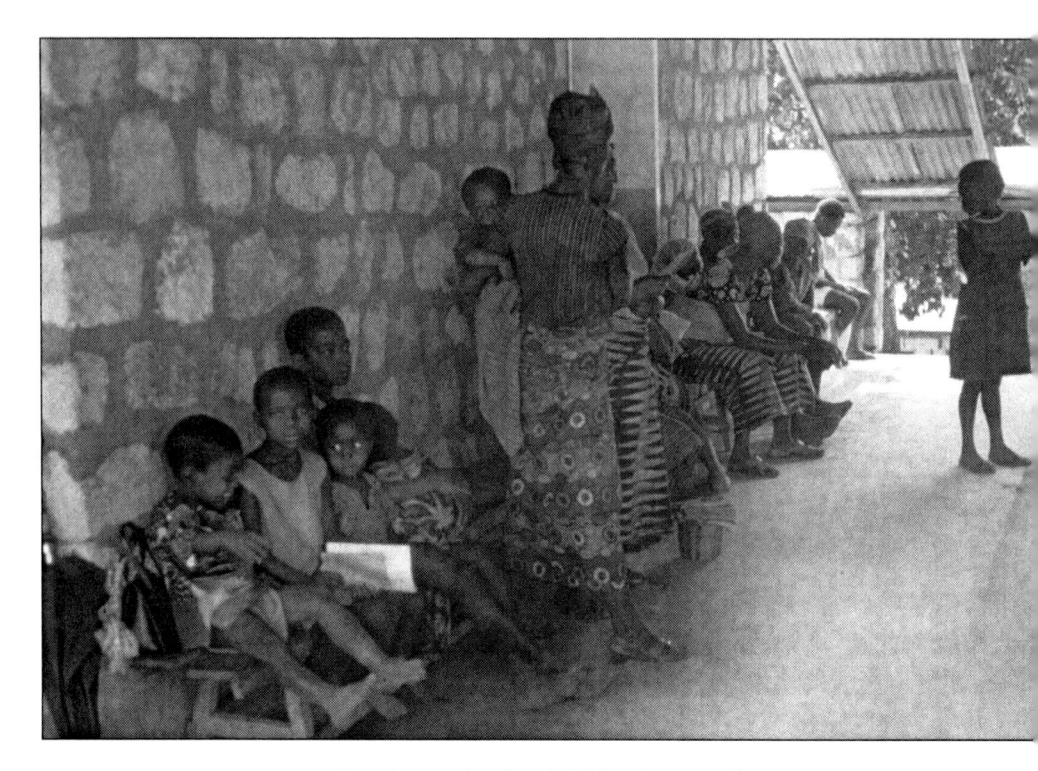

Morning mothers' and children's waiting line

When I left Cameroon, and Africa, my students presented me with two gifts. One was a set of native robe and cap, embroidered in the bright colors, red and orange and yellow and green and black, of West Africa.

The other was a carved plaque, of local wood, about two by three feet. On its front side were trees, and beasts, and people. On the back side, in black magic marker, each of the students had written their names. And in the middle of the names, in blue magic marker, was the phrase, "Seek the True Service of Medicine."

I was all the more proud, since I had never spoken those words to them, and yet they had left, in that wonderful ambiguous African way, either a compliment to me which I scarce deserved, or, more likely, a testament to their own aspirations.

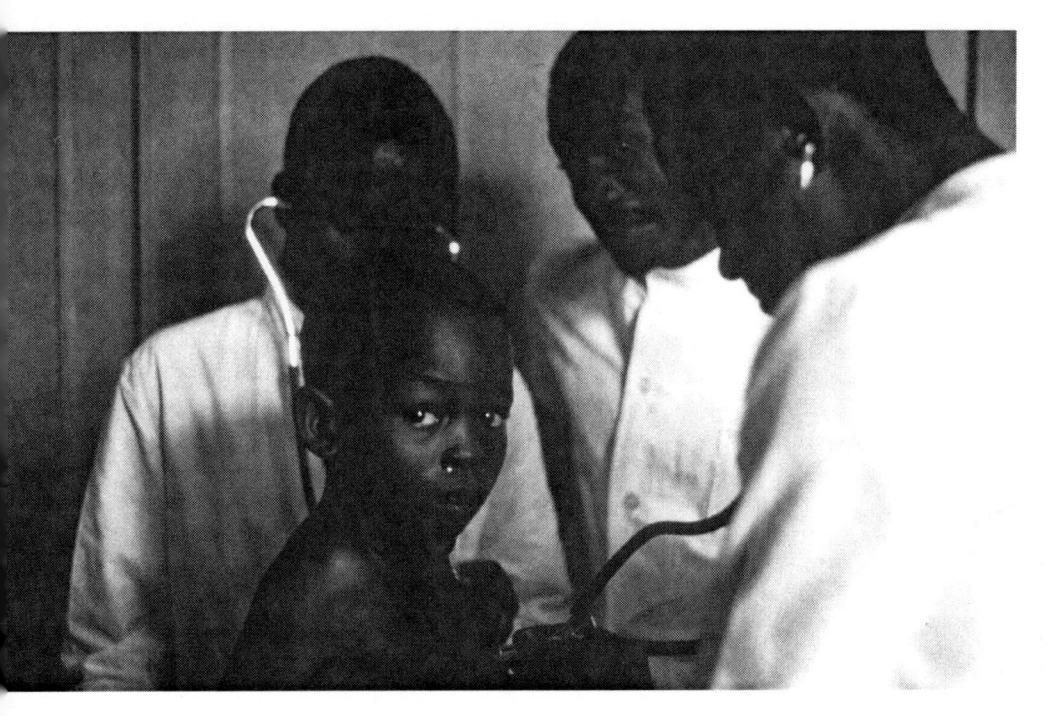

The next generation

9

Though the *Hôpital Central* and the CUSS were the largest single elements of my time in West Africa, there were a number of other activities that made the experience all the richer. Chief among these were my relationships with the French physicians and the remnants of the colonial health services, my other work for USAID in the surrounding countries, some unorthodox traveling, and my "extra-curricular" or "side-practice" of medicine, similar to that which I had undertaken in Nepal.

It seems a timeless certainty that the Americans and the French are oil on water. Ambivalence personified, repelling and attracting, sharing and sniping, unable to let go of their fascination for one another and yet equally unable to prevent a strange antipathy from surfacing and re-surfacing.

What I found in Yaoundé was that much of this was generation-related. Most of the older French, those who had been adults before or during the Second World War, would in general refuse to speak English, smile snidely at my efforts to speak French, view me as an interloper in their lost Colonial Paradise Empire, and be sure to take every opportunity to point out the bumptious ignorance and naivete of everything American. Perhaps, I thought, it was their defensive reaction to their own painful realization that, largely but for us, they would all be speaking German. You see, there I go, just like all the other Yanks.

But the younger ones, particularly the young physicians with whom I worked, and their families, were quite different, or perhaps it was that I behaved differently with them. I found that you had to work hard at it, and carefully, and pay due deference to *la belle France,* but when you broke through, you had friends worth having. And the truth is, the French and their beautiful country have many virtues, and much to admire. You also learned the other name that the French have for us: *'les Amis'*, compound slang for 'Americans' and 'friends'.

Even though a decade after independence the health services of the West African countries were titularly under African national control, in actuality the French still ruled the roost in many ways. The major hospitals depended on French *coopérants* for much of their specialty medical services. Even more so, the rural mobile clinical and public health services were at that time still run directly by the French *Médicins Militaires*, the remnants of the old military colonial mobile services, now operating under the thin guise of "regional" cooperative organizations serving the former colonies of West and Central Francophone Africa.

I found them fascinating, romantic, shades of a bit of *Beau Geste*. And besides, these guys really knew their business, had been roving Africa for years, decades some of them, and had a fund of experience, knowledge, and wild and wooly stories that was well worth paying attention to.

The head of the Central Africa Mobile Public Health Services (though that is not the actual translation, it will suffice), based in Yaoundé, was General Rene LaBouteillier. Aptly named, he was said to own a vineyard chateau in Bourgogne, and his map-veined nose attested to it. Imperious, aloof, scornful of upstart juvenile Americans. He would look down at you across his purple proboscis, over his ample belly, and sort of sniffle at you. We tried to engage his organization in some way in the teaching program of the CUSS, which would have been extremely valuable, but General LaBouteillier wasn't having anything to do with this *faux* medical school. "*Merci, et adieu, Mon General!*"

But his younger Deputy, Dr. (Colonel) Bernard Reynard, was another cat (or fox) entirely. Tough little guy, from Marseilles, looked to be right off the docks. An unlit *Gallois* hanging perpetually off the corner of the lower lip. Raspy Provencal voice. Slang—*mec, gars, paff, sac' bleu*—the whole deal. But a sharp mind, and a demon for talking and teaching about what he knew of Africa, and if the General never shared his wine, Bernard was always good for a *'Trente-Trois'* beer after work. His wife was a vision of aristocratic elegance and charm, soft-voiced, and four inches taller than he was. What more could you ask for than a rowdy New Year's

Eve with the Reynards and their younger friends in an outdoor café under the trees? Good company and laughter are at home in any language. I can do a pretty good imitation of the Fox, and I surely learned a lot of colorful and naughty words from him, but cartoon character he was not, most definitely. Good man.

The Mutt and Jeff French *coopérant* clinicians I worked with at the CUSS were of the same breed of Gallic logical competence. Pierre was an academic internist, a bit pedantic perhaps, but with a twinkle in his eye. Short and round, he didn't think much of all this public health stuff, but he knew how to run a hospital service, and how to teach on it. His wife, Germaine, the family spark plug, was a delicately-boned dermatologist who had an upscale Paris practice in Neuilly at the American Hospital. She was one-quarter Vietnamese, and had grown up in Senegal where she and Pierre had met when he came to teach at the medical school there. She took delight, a delight she communicated to her little girls, in things American, as if it was some comic-book sparkling world.

Jean-Claude was cool and collected where Pierre was hot and peppery. He was tall and lean, stooped slightly, with the look of a busy and chronically fatigued general surgeon. He had a sardonic sense of humor, and was deadly serious about his work. His wife, Claudine, was quiet, indrawn a bit, the daughter of a well-known medical professor in Marseilles where both she and Jean-Claude were from.

Our friendships lasted for many years, and if they have lapsed, it was because of my own characteristic inattention, and not theirs. My children went to them in France over the years, and theirs visited me in New York. On the many occasions that I saw Pierre and Germaine in Paris I was always welcomed in their home and felt as if only a day or two had passed since the last visit.

If the above sounds like a bit of fluff, let me illustrate what these two men were capable of by describing one of the more extraordinary efforts I have ever seen a physician put forth.

Pierre phoned me one Sunday evening. "Steve, can you come over to the hospital and give us a hand? Jean-Claude and I need a bit of help."

A French tourist, enjoying the tropical beach down at Kribi on the

Atlantic coast, had been stricken with a sudden paralysis of his left leg, and was now having trouble breathing. He was taken a hundred miles by bush taxi up to Yaoundé to the *Hôpital Central*, and Pierre, the ranking internist, was called to see him. It seemed likely that he had acute poliomyelitis which was rife in Kribi. The spinal tap supported the diagnosis, and the affliction was spreading rapidly upward to impede his chest muscles.

Pierre called Jean-Claude. The hospital had no mechanical ventilators of any sort. So Pierre and Jean-Claude took up an Ambu Bag, a volley-ball-sized springy hollow rubber ball with mouth/nose mask attached at one end, and a connector for a tube that can lead to an oxygen cylinder at the other. The Ambu is what is used on ambulances and in emergency rooms and such, for temporarily assisting ventilation while stabilizing or reviving a patient. The attendant squeezes the bag, pushing air rhythmically into the patient's lungs through the mask. One's hand tires quickly; the effort is similar to the exercise of squeezing a rubber ball. Ten minutes seems a very long time.

By the time I got there, Pierre and Jean-Claude had been at it for several hours, taking turns, the one who was "off" the bag doing the other chores necessary to care for the patient. Meanwhile, the patient had become unconscious, and the paralysis of his respiratory muscles was now virtually total, as the disease moved upward, also affecting the respiratory centers in the brain stem.

Obviously, they could use a third pair of hands so I pitched in and we rotated the squeeze every five or ten minutes. I asked them what their plans were for keeping the guy alive.

"*Eh, mon vieux*," grunted Pierre as he squeezed the bag, "*Pas difficile. Je vais lui transporter vers Paris.*" ("Simple, old chap. I'm going to move him to Paris.")

"Paris! How the hell are you going to get him to Paris? It's a seven-hour flight, and the plane doesn't go until tomorrow, late morning, and there is no mechanical ventilator either here or in flight."

"*Calme-toi, mon ami*," put in Jean-Claude from the other side of the gurney that they had the patient laid out on, "*On va faire le bulot, 'vec toi, jusqu'à demain matin, et, alors, Pierre va jouer au " volleyball" et ils vont arriver à Paris.*" ("Relax, buddy, we'll take care of it, with you, until tomorrow morning, and then Pierre is going to play volleyball and they will make it to Paris.")

And that's exactly what happened. They arranged for a litter and six empty seats, two abreast, on the UAL morning flight to Paris. I helped them through the night. We kept the patient going and in the morning we loaded him, while squeezing the Ambu all the while, into Jean-Claude's Peugeot 504 station wagon and took him to the airport. It took all three of us to get the litter and the patient up the stairs and into the plane, bagging all the way. And then Pierre, all by himself, just squeezed that black Ambu bag all the way across the Sahara to Paris, seven hours or more, and was met by an ambulance at Charles de Gaulle airport. Say, twenty squeezes per minute, times eight hours, or a steady nine and a half thousand squeezes, all by himself. I expect he couldn't even get a cabin attendant to spell him so that he could go to the bathroom. I'll bet Pierre couldn't hold a cigarette, let alone strike a match, or button his buttons, for a week.

The patient lived, and actually made a full recovery, so he could still go and swim at the beach.

✦ ✦ ✦

One of the most painful episodes of my medical life concerned my dear friends Jean-Claude and Claudine. They asked me to examine Annabelle, their two-year old daughter, about whose development they were concerned.

The child sat on the edge of the examining table, seemingly in a world of her own. Annabelle's limbs and motor activity were strong and symmetrical, but she would not walk. She rocked back and forth, humming and whispering unintelligibly to herself, and not responding in any noticeable way to attempts to communicate with her, though simple testing made it clear her sight and hearing were normal. At intervals she would give a shrill cry, and twist about. But the fundamental movement was the rocking, and what her mother described as head-banging against her crib slats at home. There were no localizing signs that would point to a structural neurologic defect.

The diagnosis seemed clear, even to my inexpert examination: infantile autism. Cause: completely unknown. Therapy: non-existent. Prognosis at the time: hopeless for amelioration or cure. I suggested that Jean-Claude and Claudine consult a specialist when they went on home leave to Marseilles in a few months. They returned from France without Annabelle who was left in the care of her grandmother and eventually institutionalized.

I suppose that my friends' tragedy was no different than so many of the tragedies that I dealt with daily on my wards, but it seemed so arbitrary, so cruel to all the lives involved, and so much closer to my own life, that it struck me deeply, and has stayed with me. I have never encountered another patient in whom I made a fresh diagnosis of autism.

✦ ✦ ✦

I continued to make occasional visits to Bangui, the capital city of the Central African Republic, learning more about the country and seeing if there might be any opening to work with the government on a health center expansion project. It was slow going.

One Christmas my family and I decided to drive overland from Yaoundé to Bangui, a distance of six or seven hundred miles. I cranked up the VW Camper Bus and my wife, my two young daughters, the Lion Dog, and I set out.

The road was mostly paved the first hundred miles or so as it was the only land route from the coast of West Africa to Bangui in the east and also to Fort Lamy, Chad, in the north. At N'gaoundere in northern Cameroon the routes divided and we turned southeast towards Bangui in the Central African Republic.

Now we were on the dusty (at least at that season, but muddy beyond belief in the spring and summer) red laterite dirt roads of Africa, passing through dry bush with the occasional small thatched village. Save for the road bisecting it, the landscape must have looked very much the same a thousand years ago.

About 25 miles beyond N'gaoundere, in the middle of nowhere, the VW suddenly lost power. After skidding to a stop (the dry-season laterite dust is as slick as the rainy-season mud is sticky), I realized that I had no forward traction in any gear, but that I could "advance" in reverse. This suggested a burned-out clutch. The next isolated small town was about fifty miles ahead beyond the frontier into the Central African Republic. It was impractical to turn the vehicle around and then "back up" fifty miles, but remembering that we had passed a tiny village about six or seven miles back, I thought that might be a reasonable target. If we could get some kind of shelter or help there we would be still within Cameroon and only fifteen miles or so from N'gaoundere where there were government posts and a railroad line back to Yaoundé. If I needed to order automobile parts or send my family back to Yaoundé, I could do it from N'gaoundere.

So we put her into reverse and slowly and carefully backed up the six miles into the village of no name, a collection of fifteen or twenty thatched huts and nothing else. As we arrived, the villagers clustered around to greet us, and then the crowd parted as a tall, dignified man in a long robe and cap approached. His French was only slightly better than my own.

"What is your difficulty, and how can my village help you?" When I explained the situation, he paused thoughtfully for a moment, and then spoke again. "You can probably get a ride on one of the trucks that pass along the road towards N'gaoundere. Your family and your dog will be safe here; we will take good care of them. In N'gaoundere you can arrange for some way to repair your car, or to transport your family back to Yaoundé. Do not worry, I am the chief here, and I will set my own son to guard your vehicle."

It seemed like the best alternative and so, thanking him, I stood out on the road with my thumb stuck out while my family was shepherded into the village. Because this was the overland truck route, it was only a matter of fifteen or twenty minutes before a huge Berliot *camion* squealed to a halt in a choking cloud of red dust, and within the hour I was dropped off at the N'gaoundere *Préfet's* (District Officer's) quarters. It being a Sunday, my obliging truck driver combed the town until we found the place.

The *Préfet* listened to my story, and said, "The District Hospital here in N'gaoundere has some VW vans, and perhaps they will have the spare part that you need. Since it is late Sunday afternoon, I suggest that we wait until morning to see what can be done. There is a monastery here in N'gaoundere and I am sure that the Brothers there will give you and your family shelter for tonight. I will send my Jeep and driver with you now back out to the village to collect your family and bring you all back here. Then tomorrow we can see what is possible and, if nothing else, you can go back by train or send your family back to Yaoundé, order the spare part there, or whatever makes most sense."

Less than an hour later, I was back in the village in the middle of nowhere. A small boy of about eight years was proudly standing guard, ramrod straight, over the VW by the side of the road. I found my family in the chief's hut, sitting on the floor among a crowd of women and children, to whom the Lion Dog and my youngest daughter's blondish hair seemed to be the chief topics of amusement and conversation. I explained the plan to the chief, who insisted that his son would stand guard all night, and that I should not worry.

And so, less than an hour later again, we were in the whitewashed monastery at N'gaoundere, where the African and French Brothers fed and housed us with true hospitality.

On Monday morning, I walked over to the District Hospital, and introduced myself to the *Médicin Chef*. "It is your good fortune," he said, "that there happens to be in N'gaoundere a fine mechanic trained at the Volkswagen depot in Yaoundé. He lives outside town and I will have to send for him, but if you will come back here this afternoon we will see what we can do."

I had heard the stories about African bush mechanics who can fix anything with match-sticks and electrician's tape (and sometimes without the tape), but I was somewhat skeptical. When I arrived back at the hospital in the early afternoon, there he was, a lanky fellow in tattered shorts and once-white tee shirt and torn tennis shoes. He said, "*Sprechen Zie Deutch?*" (Speak German?). When I replied, "No, but it goes in French," and told him what had happened, he said, "Sounds like a worn clutch-plate, all right. We have no spares."

My face fell, then he continued, "But we do have a broken down VW bus standing out in the yard, and its clutch plate is probably serviceable.

Tell you what, we can take the clutch-plate out of that vehicle, take it to the village, use it to replace yours, and then you can go on your way to Bangui. There is a VW dealer there. They can put in a new clutch-plate, give you mine back, and then when you pass through N'gaoundere on your journey home to Yaoundé, you can give return it to me. How's that sound?"

He removed the clutch-plate from the VW, which stood up on cement blocks with tall grass growing out of the sunroof, and, once again, within the hour of collecting mechanic, clutch-plate, wife, children, and dog, we again arrived by Jeep at the village. The young guard was still on duty.

Now the clutch on the old VW Camper Bus is in the rear with the motor, and not so easy to get at. It was now almost dark, and I was dismayed to see that the mechanic could not reach as far as he needed to change plates. "Not to worry, " he said, and conferred briefly with the chief. Within minutes, ten men appeared, carrying between them several kerosene lanterns and a log about ten feet long and six inches in diameter. The lanterns were lit, the log placed under the rear of the chassis from side to side, with five men on each end, everybody said, "Hup-Ah!" and lifted the rear end of the bus off the ground, and held it there. The mechanic calmly crawled under, disengaged the faulty plate, crawled out again to give everyone a rest, then "Hup-Ah!" again, and he repeated the procedure, this time installing the new plate. He refused payment, but I stuck some Central African francs in what remained of his shirt pocket, and he and the Jeep were on their way south to N'gaoundere, and we prepared to spend the night in our Camper Bus a few miles down the road toward Bangui.

I tried to give some money to the chief, "For the village." He refused, waving me off. "You were a traveler in difficulty in my village," he said. "It is my duty and my honor to help you, and my son's obligation to see that no harm came to your vehicle. I cannot take any payment from you. May Allah see to it that the rest of your journey be smooth, and may we meet again."

The clutch worked fine, and we made the rest of the trip to Bangui uneventfully, including a Christmas Eve overnight stop at a Central African

Republic Young Pioneers' Camp, where, as usual, the wonders of the camper bus and the Lion Dog assured us of a warm, if not hilarious, welcome from the Young Pioneers. In Bangui, it was a matter of an hour for the VW agency to switch clutch-plates again. They, however, had a hydraulic lift. We spent a few days in Bangui, where the atmosphere of government paranoia was matched by the best-ever *beignets* and coffee at the local bakery, and chugged back to Yaoundé across the grasslands and through the savanna, and down across the forest. In Bangui, we had bought several bolts of brightly-colored cloth for the women of "our village," and bags of candy for the children (including the intrepid sentinel). The chief seemed genuinely moved and we shook hands in the French African way, with the left hand clasping the right shoulder as the right hands clasped each other, after which the right hand briefly touched one's own heart.

We gave the *Médicin Chef's* old clutch plate back to him, found that the mechanic had disappeared back off into the bush, and thanked the Brothers at the monastery for their hospitality. I realized why I loved Africa.

✦ ✦ ✦

But of the places in Africa that I knew, it was Chad that fascinated me most. It was off the map, the variety of its vast interior stretching from the wetlands and savanna of the south, through the progressively drier Sahel at the center, on to the true Sahara in the north. In the south, you could still watch massive crocodiles slithering along the mud-banks of the rivers and troops of elephants crashing through the bush. It was a world that seemed to me little changed from that described by Romain Gary in his decades-past novel, *The Roots of Heaven*. In the center, once you left Fort Lamy, you were in the true bush, tiny thatched villages surrounded by fields of sorghum and millet, connected by foot-paths and the wandering dirt track.

Further north, you would encounter the occasional nomadic band, herding their goats and long-horned cattle through the dry thornbush and parched grasses. I never was able to travel to the true north, the true desert, the true Sahara, and have always regretted it.

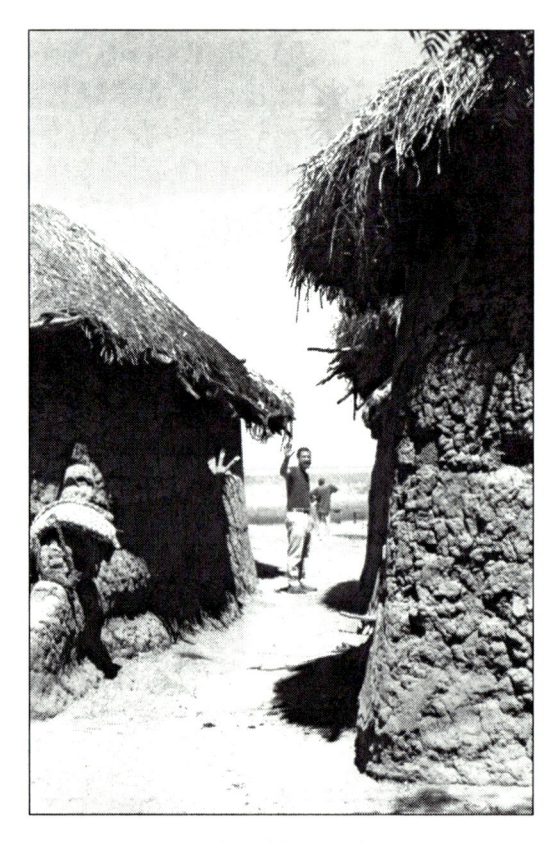

Edge of the Sahel

Once I was in Fort Lamy during a State Visit by French President Pompidou, and all the tribes from north and south seemed to be gathered there as well, for a spectacular two days of celebration and dancing. There were naked men with spears from the southern grasslands, their bodies marked out with daubs of white clay, standing immobile, one leg bent up against the other thigh, like storks, leaning on their spears. There were villagers completely covered in tent-like cloaks of raffia, fantastic wooden masks strapped atop their heads, small drums and rattles in their hands. There were the wandering N'doboro and Tubu in sandals, flowing robes, and wide, shallow conical straw hats, daggers strapped inside their sleeves, their faces painted like porcelain dolls with white and red and yellow around their eyes and mouths, and choreographed staccato gestures that made them look like puppets held on strings. There were the horsemen from the north, with ancient long muskets and sabers who, in the traditional *fantasia* would come swooping and galloping down the parade ground with wild cries, firing their muskets and screaming as they rode full tilt. And there were the true nomads of the north, the Blue People, the Tuareg, clothed and stained in indigo, their faces covered by a turban-end, as silent and self-possessed as their camels.

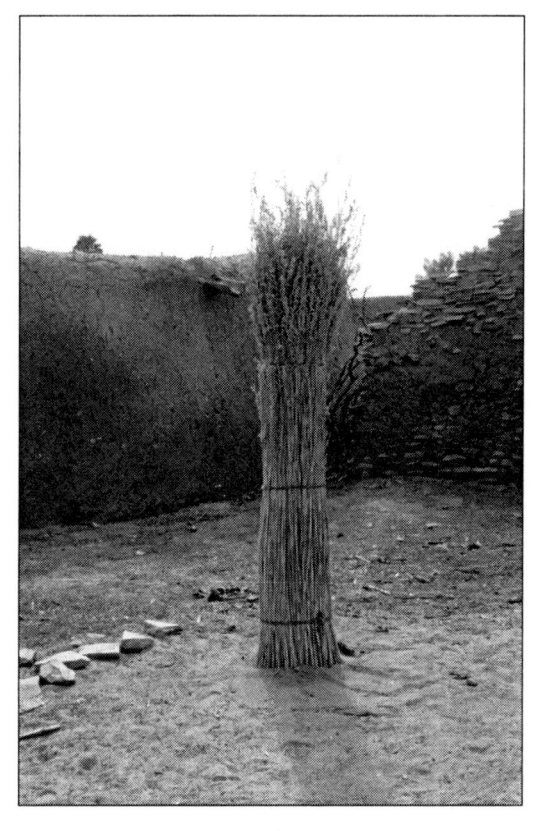

In a good year...

In quieter times Fort Lamy had a mysterious beauty, a sleepy dusty town, sun blazing fiercely at mid-day, moon immense at night, the muddy

Chari flowing nearby, in its corridor of rushes and small trees, and singing birds. The Hotel Chadienne sat alongside the river, *blancs* and a few *noirs* drinking and talking softly on the veranda by the pool, under the infinite black dome of the sky. During the month long holy days of Ramadan when the Faithful take neither food nor drink from sunrise to sunset, the town was silent, the air still, a few white-robed figures immobile in the scarce shade of walls or the thin trees of the central plazas, seeking relief from the searing sun, and waiting impassively for dusk, and water, some going all day without swallowing their saliva.

Until the cholera came, my work in Chad didn't amount to much: seeing to the completion of a health center on the edge of town that USAID had funded and negotiating the shape of an expanded program of rural health with Dr. Bondo, with whom my friendship deepened. To be honest, these were as much excuses for me to travel to and around Chad as anything else.

✦ ✦ ✦

Back in Yaoundé, in addition to my work at the hospital and at the CUSS, I also had the leavening of an informal practice among the Americans and other expatriates, much as I had had in Nepal.

One Sunday evening (the time when medical problems arise disproportionately) I got a call from the American Ambassador.

"Steve, could you come have a look at Terry (his twelve year old daughter)? She has had a severe bellyache all day, but no diarrhea, and is now vomiting repeatedly."

When I examined her, the diagnosis was no more difficult than it had been years earlier up on the Tibetan Frontier. Waiting for evacuation to France or to the U.S. military hospital in Germany was out of the question. But fortunately, this time there was a *real* surgeon available. I asked Jean-Claude to see the girl, and two hours later we were in the operating room at *Hôpital Central*, me watching how a pro did it instead of sweating through the appendectomy myself. Jean-Claude did a quick job, the parents were suitably impressed, and from that point forward, if there was anything at all that the CUSS needed from the Americans, we got it.

Early in my time in Cameroun, I got a call from the manager of the Mont Febe Palace Hotel, up on the mountain outside of town. Would I have a look at his wife who seemed to have trouble walking?

They were an attractive and very young couple. He was French, she was Croatian. Previously in good general health, and without a recent minor illness, she had been experiencing a weakness in both legs for two or three days which seemed to be getting worse. On examining her, she had no changes in sensation, no pain, and a symmetrical weakness of both legs. I could find no other neurological abnormalities, and her mental status was clear and completely normal.

She claimed to have been immunized in childhood against polio, but I was fairly confident that this was not polio. What it fit closely was a syndrome known as Guillain-Barre, which classically comprised a symmetric ascending paralysis without sensory or other changes. Guillain-Barre Syndrome is not an actively infectious disease, but rather some sort of immunologic response to an unknown precursor, perhaps an infection. A spinal tap shows an inflammatory reaction, with increased levels of protein and cells characteristic of a chronic inflammatory response. This strange disease is self-limited, and usually leaves no permanent disability, But in some cases it can progress upwards far enough to impair, or prevent, breathing. Thus, some patients require prolonged mechanical ventilatory assistance, sometimes for weeks or even months, before the paralysis descends and disappears.

It seemed to me that I could do the spinal tap and solidify the diagnosis, ruling out other possibilities. However, I was quite sure of my diagnosis and what would the spinal tap actually achieve? Her paralysis seemed to be ascending fairly rapidly and there were no facilities to care for her adequately in Cameroon. I was confident that this was not a garden variety meningitis. If, on the other hand, it turned out not to be Guillain-Barre, but something even more obscure, I didn't know what it was, and didn't have the means to find out in Yaoundé. I decided that the most important element for her was time—time to get her to Europe for definitive diagnosis and, most importantly, before any respiratory difficulty occurred.

"Madame, it would really be best for you to leave Yaoundé for

Paris as soon as possible, by tomorrow's plane if you can." I explained my reasoning, but I had a strong suspicion that they thought I was trying to rid myself of the case, because I didn't know what I was dealing with or what to do about it.

Their reaction to me was rather stiff, but they packed hurriedly and left on the morning plane. The diagnosis turned out to be correct. She never had any respiratory difficulty and recovered fully in three weeks time, but they never returned to Yaoundé. Sometimes you do the right thing, and no-one will ever realize you did it. And then again, sometimes you do the wrong thing, and no-one will ever realize you did it.

A woman from the French Embassy brought her housemaid to see me. The young woman kept her head down and her eyes fixed on the floor.

"*Docteur*, once I had six children. All of them seemed to be perfectly healthy. *(beware when patients use that exact phrase)*, and then each died suddenly at about a year of age. I was left with no children, and now my seventh child, my little girl, is coming to her first birthday. I am very frightened, *Docteur*, and don't know what to do."

The young woman spoke French well, and I was able to question her exhaustively. There was no pattern that I could discern. No other family history of mysterious deaths or illnesses, nothing that sounded like "crib death," nothing I could recognize as a congenital malady, no history of illness in the children before they were found dead.

While she didn't want to use the word, she was obviously convinced that it was witchcraft, some kind of curse. She seemed passive and depressed, and I could tell that she was consulting me only because her French mistress insisted upon it.

I examined the child carefully, did what screening laboratory and x-ray testing I could, and found nothing abnormal. I heard or saw nothing that would make me suspect some bizarre sort of child abuse or neglect. All I could think of to say was to ask that the woman contact me immediately if the child should show any sign of illness or distress.

A month later, I got a call from the French woman. The seventh child was dead. She did not know how or exactly when, and the mother had gone back upcountry to her village.

Had I missed something? Was there anything to miss? Some of your patients stay in your mind forever.

✦ ✦ ✦

John and Emily Green were an American couple. He was a junior officer in the Information Division at the Embassy. It was his second marriage, her first, and at age thirty-four, she was delighted to discover that she was pregnant. They sat in the Embassy health room, holding hands, after I had finished examining her. I congratulated them, and said, "Everything seems to be fine. I am very happy for you, and expect that you are going to have a lovely baby. You really have two choices. You can stay here to deliver at the Central Hospital, where facilities are not the best, but where there is an excellent British-trained Cameroonian obstetrician, or you can go up to Germany, to the U.S. military hospital at Wiesbaden, several months before your due date, and be delivered there.

They looked at each other, and then at me. "Doctor, I'm not leaving," she said. "John and I want to be together for this, and we are going to have our baby here. Under no circumstances am I leaving Yaoundé."

"Okay, that seems like a sensible choice as long as everything is alright, which it seems to be. I'll be at your delivery, for sure, and take care of the baby. Let me give you a referral now to Dr. Nasah, and he can take it from there. I'll keep in touch with him as things go along. You'll like Dr. Nasah (and I knew they would) and he is fully-trained and very competent."

Bernie Nasah, my colleague at the CUSS and *Hôpital Central,* was a West Cameroonian, well-trained and very conscientious, and I had full confidence in him. Pediatricians and Obstetricians tend to look each other over very carefully.

A month or so later, Bernie pulled me aside one morning, while I was making rounds at the hospital.

"Steve. Emily Green. Well, you know, she's thirty-four, a first pregnancy, and she does have a rather narrow pelvic outlet, nothing too restricted. But the point is, she's carrying twins. Do you really think she should deliver here?"

I sat down with the Greens.

"Emily, it's just that the risk of trouble is always multiplied by all the factors, any one of which by itself is not necessarily of great concern. This is your first pregnancy, you don't have what we would call a "proven pelvis," you're a little older than mostly all first mothers, and you're carrying twins. Dr. Nasah and I have talked, and we think it might be better if you went up to Europe, or home to the States if you wanted, to have the babies. Not that we really expect any difficulty, but, you know . . . "

"Dr. Joseph, Steve, I am having my babies right here. John and I want to be together for this. We have talked about it, and our minds are made up."

"Emily, John, I am sure that I could convince the Ambassador to give John special leave to be with you in Germany for a few weeks before and after the births. You would only be separated for a short time. I really think it would be best, but it is, of course, your decision."

"We are staying. Period."

I admired them, in a way. Bernie and I came up with a plan. One of our CUSS colleagues, a French professor of physiology, had married a Cameroonian woman who had been trained in France as a nurse-midwife. Genevieve was from a wealthy urbanized Ewondo family and had set herself up in a private maternity clinic in town not far from the railway station. Bernie had worked with her before and judged that the clinic was far cleaner and better equipped than his own facilities at *Hôpital Central*. So when the time came, he would deliver Emily Green at Genevieve's clinic and I would be there to deal with the twins.

The pregnancy went along uneventfully, and just about at her due date, early one Monday morning, Emily Green went into labor. I got to the clinic about seven-thirty and she had already been in labor for about five hours. She was in a comfortable bed in a small but neat room, next door to the delivery room which was also spotlessly clean and seemed well equipped.

"Nothing is moving fast here," noted Bernie. "Why don't you go over and make rounds and come back in a couple of hours. I can get a message to you at the hospital if anything comes up."

Not having heard from Bernie, I got back over to the clinic a little before noon, thinking I would have a look in, and then go home for a quick lunch. After all, she had only been in labor about 9 or 10 hours, her water hadn't broken as far as I knew, and that was pretty much par for the course for a first-timer.

Genevieve met me at the door of the clinic, worry evident on her face. "Steve, Bernie was just going to call you. We need to talk about this."

Bernie was as calm as always, but evidently concerned. "She's not progressing very well at all. Dilation hasn't moved for a couple of hours now. Her water broke a few minutes ago, and the fluid was meconium-stained (evidence of fetal distress). Let's give it a little longer, but if things don't progress rapidly, we have to think about a Caesarian."

I went to see Emily, who looked strained but not unduly so. She smiled thinly when I told her that the fetal heartbeat, or rather heartbeats, sounded good to me. I also told her that she had better hurry up because I had a tennis game scheduled for later in the afternoon.

Over the next two hours, she didn't progress. When Bernie on one of his regular checks heard a fetal heartbeat slowing, we knew it was decision time. Obstetrics has been defined somewhere as long hours of boredom punctuated by minutes of white-knuckled terror. When things start to go wrong, it seems they often cascade from bad to worse very rapidly. I wondered whether I should have argued harder for Emily to deliver in Europe, and I knew that the answer was yes.

"Okay," said Genevieve, "I'll get things ready in there."

Genevieve was terrific. She managed light drip anesthesia much better than I could have. Bernie had her prepped in no time, and before I knew it he was in the belly, through the uterus, and pulling out the first twin, which he handed off to me while he cut and tied the cord, and went back for the second baby.

The boy was good-sized for a twin, and well-formed. The trouble was that he was limp, blue, and not breathing. Sometimes C-section babies are a little slow that way since they don't have their lungs squeezed as they come through the birth canal, but this was clearly different. Laid on the countertop along the wall, he was a dish-rag, not responding to physical stimulation, so I cleaned out his pharynx with a manual suction device, put the tiny Ambu bag over his nose and mouth, and started to give him gentle puffs of oxygen from the tank that Genevieve had connected to the Ambu. With my forefinger I felt for the pulse, which was weak and a bit slow, but steady. His color came up a bit, but there was still no spontaneous respiration or movement or attempt to cry. Just as I was getting my thoughts organized as to what to do next, Bernie shouted at me.

"Steve, get over here, and get the second one. He's not breathing, and I have to get the placenta out, she's leaking blood like a sieve."

I pushed Genevieve at the first baby, knowing she knew what to do to continue bagging him, and grabbed the second from Bernie. Part of my mind registered the fact that these were two boys with one placenta, identical twins, how lovely.

The second twin was, if anything, more depressed than his older brother. Not breathing, limp, poor color, heart rate and rhythm so-so. I suctioned him out, putting a different catheter tip on the sucker, and started to give him gentle mouth-to-mouth, since we only had one Ambu. Just as I could feel him give a few tiny respiratory efforts of his own, Genevieve called out, "Steve, the first one's heart has stopped!"

You know the old expression, "Never rains but it pours"? That's how it generally is when things go sour in the delivery room. I switched babies with Genevieve. I moved over to the first twin, felt no heartbeat, saw no chest wall movement. Picking up the neonatal laryngoscope that we probably wouldn't have had in the *Hôpital Central*, I put a catheter down his windpipe and sucked it out clean (there was meconium-stained fluid deep down), slid in a tiny endotracheal tube (thank God I was lucky enough to get it in right the first time; that has not always been easy for me with newborns), grabbed the Ambu back from Genevieve, and gave him a few gentle puffs of oxygen.

But his heart still wasn't beating. "How's Twin Two doing, Genevieve?"

"Seems all right. Breathing on his own, heart rate is good, color's coming up, and even gave a little cry a moment ago. He's going to be all right, I think. Let me just clean him off and wrap him in a blanket."

"Just cover him, don't clean him, we can do that later. Get over here and help me with this one."

"What the hell is going on over there?" said Bernie, whom I had never heard say even "darn" before. "I'll be finished closing here in a couple of minutes and then can help you two. Emily's okay, pulse and color good, beginning to come up to the surface."

After turning the Ambu over to Genevieve, I gave Twin One a few quick chest compressions to try and get his heart going, then broke open a vial of epinephrine, drew up a tiny bit into a syringe, and injected it directly through the chest wall into his heart. Perhaps I was a bit premature in doing that, maybe should have worked at closed chest massage a little longer, but I thought we had better pull all the stops out, given how things had gone.

Somehow, the three or four minutes that had passed since Bernie handed me the first baby, and that had seemed like hours, resolved themselves into real time, and everything began to swim into place. I don't remember all the evolution, but in about five more minutes we had two pink babies, lying on their mother's breast, wrapped in thin cotton blankets. I remember that one had cried lustily, and most satisfactorily, during the process, but I don't remember which one it was. Emily was half-awake, and whispered drunkenly to me, "See, I knew I should do it here."

I suddenly remembered John, outside in the labor room, whose last awareness had been when we rushed Emily into the delivery room. I went out to see him, sitting rigid on Emily's bed, staring at nothing.

"I heard a lot of noise in there. Is everything all right? Is Emily all right?"

"Emily and your two big boys are fine, John, fine. Sometimes things move a little quickly, but everything is A-okay now." (I prayed silently that the twins had weathered the storm, and that there would be no unpleasant surprises with their development in the weeks and months ahead.) Why don't you go in now and see them."

While the two of them, or I should say the four of them, embraced, Bernie and Genevieve and I just looked at each other, letting our heart rates come down and our thoughts settle, not knowing how to put that frantic

193

lifetime into words. Then Genevieve said, "Let me get them all tucked away, and let's the three of us have a beer."

About seventeen years later, out of the blue, I received a letter with a Vermont return address. Before I could read the letter itself, a color photograph fell out of the envelope. It showed a middle-aged couple, looking very Vermontish, backed by green hills and a cabin. They were standing between two massive young men, six-two or -three at least, who towered over their parents. Everyone had their arms around each other, and everyone was smiling.

It doesn't get any better than that. Ever.

10

Have you ever watched some phenomenon of nature coming toward you through the distance, moving steadily, sometimes in slow-motion, inexorably, with a decisiveness seldom seen in purely human affairs? Say, a rising surf-line before an ocean storm or hurricane, or a broken line of squalls all across your frontal vision, under the thunderheads of a desert sky?

That same sense gripped me in the early years of the 1970s, as I followed the extraordinary progress of the epidemic wave of cholera moving westward from Asia into and through the Middle East. When cholera broke out from its traditional homeland in the river estuaries of Bangladesh and moved westward across the sub-continent, into the Gulf and the Arabian peninsula, throughout the late 1960s, it was not unusual. Cholera had been doing that periodically for as long as we had studied the behavior of cholera.

This was a new strain of cholera, labeled the "El Tor," and as it moved slowly westwards abetted by the pilgrims visiting Mecca from the Middle East and North Africa, there was initially really nothing unusual in its behavior. Even when cholera pushed strongly into Iran and west along the North African coast, it was somewhat atypical but not unheard of. The tidal movements of cholera epidemics flowing and ebbing from Bangladesh had always formed an erratic, but basic, rhythmic pattern.

But then El Tor did something totally unexpected, something never before seen. It rounded the North African coast, moved south along the bulge of West Africa, and then the epidemic, in 1971 and 1972, actually flowed eastward along the African coastline, and even moved inward from the coast into the forested and dry hinterlands.

This pattern, and this disease, had never before been observed in West Africa. From my little nook of the world in Yaoundé I followed, as if running my fingers across a map, the progress of this extraordinary phenomenon, week by week, on the pages of the *International Herald Tribune*, which arrived regularly by air from Paris though several days behind schedule. Cholera cases were reported in the Spanish Sahara, in the Gambia, Senegal, Sierra Leone, and now in Nigeria, which shared its eastern border with Cameroon and Chad.

It was apparent that the cholera organisms were seeding their way in along the riverine estuaries of the West African coast, finding new habitat from which they were unlikely to ever be extirpated, new homelands for an ancient disease. Some of the most explosive outbreaks were not in the coastal cities, but in the drier lands of the interior. And from where cholera seemed to be concentrating in Nigeria, it was clear to me that the forward path of the epidemic pointed into Chad.

I was due, in any case, to visit Fort Lamy to talk with Dr. Watel Bondo about progress of the health center extension program we were trying to get off the ground. The rumors of cholera appearing in Central Chad that reached me in Yaoundé seemed to be a major reason to accelerate my visit. I knew cholera as a terrible disease, perhaps the most fulminant of epidemics, but I knew it only from what I had been taught and what I had read in the tropical disease texts. I had never seen a case. I knew there was a partially-effective vaccine, had vaccinated many people against cholera and had myself been vaccinated. I knew that there was no specific treatment that could be effectively applied en masse to a threatened or affected population. Most cholera epidemics, especially as they occurred in impoverished and unsanitary communities, just had to burn themselves out.

Arriving in Fort Lamy, I found Dr. Bondo in a state of feverish activity; for the first time lacking the equanimity and cool resolve I had come to associate with him.

"Steve, we are beginning to see increasing numbers of cases along the central frontier with Nigeria, skipping and jumping from village to village in remote areas. I have only a few physicians and nurses, short supplies of vaccine, and my plan is to try and build a *cordon sanitaire* fifty or so kilometers back from the frontier, consisting of crude field treatment stations and whatever vaccine we can bring to bear. If you would like to come with me tomorrow, I'm going up by helicopter to the zone that we think will be the initial focus of the epidemic in Chad, and can show you the situation."

The next morning, I joined Watel and a few senior Chadian military officers. We were flown in two French army choppers up into the area he had described. We landed in the middle of nowhere on a dusty cleared patch in the bush where Chadian troops were cutting posts and brush to build one of a series of "hospitals"—field treatment stations. These consisted of upright poles dug into the ground, with scaffolding on top that could be covered with long grass and brush to form a shaded, three-sided shelter over a floor of sand or dirt. To one side were several small military tents and huge stockpiles of fluid and tubing for intravenous administration.

That was all there was. Period. Four or five of these "hospitals" were to be spaced at intervals along a line parallel to the current front of the epidemic with a few truck-equipped mobile vaccination teams working back and forth along a line in the villages behind them. Beyond the intravenous fluids, provided by the French government, other medicines were virtually non-existent, save for what little could be spared from the scant Health Ministry hospital and health center stocks.

Dr. Bondo was determined to do what he could with what he had. He had mobilized teams of nurses from the rural health services and the central hospital in Fort Lamy and had scrounged a few doctors from the French military.

"What can you and your government do to help us, Steve?" he asked.

"Well, you have all the fluids you need. There is no way that any orthodox physical facilities can be built or improved in the time available. I will try to get the U.S. to send some vaccine and antibiotics and such, which are not likely to be very effective with regard to your major and immediate problem. But I'll tell you what, Watel. One extra body would increase your medical manpower by about twenty-five percent. If you'll have me, I'll come up here and staff one of your "hospitals" for as long as you need me."

He was glad to get the help and I was between terms at the CUSS, and figured that I could be away from Yaoundé for two or three weeks by which time the epidemic would have either burned through or burned out and by which time more medical help would arrive from the French and things would stabilize a bit. I reasoned that I would help out a friend whom I greatly admired, do some useful medical work, and experience a firestorm of infectious disease under primitive conditions.

Jake Raines and Ambassador Tubman in Fort Lamy were enthusiastic about the idea, and agreed to furnish me a four-wheel drive truck and some basic equipment. I played them and the Embassy and AID Mission back in Yaoundé off against each other as to who was supporting this endeavor and obtained what I considered to be adequate, if informal, clearance.

Returning quickly to Yaoundé, I put my professional and personal affairs in order, cobbled together some field equipment and rations from the Military Attaché at the Embassy and then went to see my French colleague and friend, Colonel Reynard, at the Regional Headquarters of the Mobile Health Services.

In his best Marseilles manner, Bernard Reynard made that Provencal gesture, half-way between a cluck and a spit, and growled, "Paff. Yanks. So you want to see what it's really all about, eh? *Alors, mon mec*, we'd be glad to push you along over the edge. I'm driving up there day after tomorrow with some vaccine and a vaccination team and you can come along with us. We'll drop you off at your "hospital." After that you're on your own."

"Thanks, Bernard. You're a good guy. For a frog and an old fox."

Our small motor convoy made the long haul up through Cameroon and into Chad. I picked up my truck and gear in Fort Lamy, barely pausing to say hi to Jake, and then rejoined Colonel Reynard as we covered the last stage up into the dry bush somewhere about a hundred kilometers north of Fort Lamy. There, on a late afternoon, they dropped me off in that same middle of nowhere on a dirt bush track a kilometer from the nearest mud and thatch village. To this day I don't know exactly where I was, or what the place was called. Bernard gave the Chadian nurses a nice fat guinea fowl that he had shot along the way, gave me a thumbs-up, and they were gone. I turned to survey what I had gotten myself into.

The field station, a three-sided lashed-up affair in a clearing hacked out of the bush, was built like the one I had seen several days earlier. In fact, it may have been the same place. A wood fire was kept constantly burning in the center between the arms of the shelter. Sandy soil brushed flat and clean formed the floor, upon which patients, already numbering about 60 when I arrived, were laid. Shallow depressions were scooped out under them into which poured the copious and watery diarrhea and vomitus that were the hallmarks of the disease. When the sand beneath them was soaked, fresh sand was scooped over it and under the patient. Bags of IV fluid were hung from the poles forming the shelter, running at extremely rapid rates into the veins of the patients.

The two Chadian nurses who were to be my colleagues introduced themselves and gave me a quick tour around. Christophe was black as night, blocky and ferocious-looking, with stubby tribal scars along both cheeks and across his forehead. He never smiled, spoke only when absolutely necessary, and had the most gentle hands I have ever seen in caring for patients. Numa was from the north, lighter-skinned, tall and with bones as thin as those of birds. He was constantly in motion, chattering to himself and others as he fluttered and swooped. Both men worked like demons attending to patients throughout the day and night, catching short snatches of sleep in their stuffy green military tent. They could thread a large-bore intravenous needle into the smallest and most collapsed veins. Sparing no effort, they took each death that we had, and there were many, as a personal affront. They spoke with me in French, and to each other in a soft and sibilant language of which I comprehended not a word. I shall never forget them, and would be proud to work with them again under any circumstances.

In those days, when we were ignorant of the use of oral rehydration solutions containing a salt and sugar mixture, the treatment of cholera was simple. You tried to pour fluids into the patient intravenously faster than the patient poured diarrhea out. All the fancy equations about rates and quantities of fluid replacement per body weight learned in medical school did not count for much out here. The rates and volumes that patients lost in copious watery diarrhea were truly amazing, and you just got the largest-caliber needles in that you could, ran the bags of fluid wide-open, and tried to stay ahead and prevent the patient dying of dehydration. We usually ran two bags of fluid at a time, with a needle in each arm, or leg, or groin, or scalp or neck vein in a small child, wherever we could put them in. It was fire-hose medicine, and sometimes we stayed far enough ahead, and sometimes we didn't.

I threw my gear into the small separate tent that Christophe and Numa insisted I take, and got to work with them. Patients were staggering in or being carried in by relatives, dropping into the sand under the shelter and we rushed to hook them up. Sometimes they died as we were putting the line in, sometimes they died within an hour or so of beginning treatment, sometimes they lasted a day, and we would think we were ahead of the game, and then they just faded away. If we could keep them going for two days, we usually pulled them through, though not always. These were tough, leathery people, but poorly-nourished and parasite-ridden to begin with. I learned that near the end of each day several French military open trucks would drive in with a load of new patients scoured from the surrounding villages. They would deliver them to us, sluice out the beds of the trucks, and haul away our day's dead to the burning pits.

This was not fine detail work, nor suitable employment for those who had difficulty with immersing themselves, literally, in shit, piss, vomit, and blood.

They kept coming, many of them barely alive. About half of them survived, staggering away, supported by relatives. The other half went to the burning pits. More adults than small children died (a phenomenon of cholera that, to my knowledge, no one has been able to satisfactorily explain), more old than young. Usually relatives accompanied them and sat by them on the sandy ground, fanning the faces of those too weak to keep the flies off, which was most of them.

By the middle of the first week, we had over a hundred patients laid out under the thatched poles at any one time, rotating in, rotating out. A huddled mass of relatives crowded together on the edges of the bush, cookfires going constantly. Many of these soon took the places of patients under the thatch; some were already infected when they arrived, some were infected as they waited in the unsanitary conditions. There was only well water from the nearby village (the nurses and I drank distilled water from the IV bags, cut open at the corner and drained like a coconut), there was no sanitation, and no way to prevent contamination. Flies in enormous numbers moved from the sick to the well, from pools of excrement to patients and relatives alike.

When a patient came in, we made a quick assessment and got to work. There was no point in attempting triage: we had one disease to combat (whatever else they had) and one therapy to employ. We pulled bags of various water, salt, and sugar solutions off the small mountain of IV fluids, put in the needles, and ran in the solution as fast as we could, tapering off in rough calculation of progress. Inflow versus outflow, that was all it was about. Twenty-four hours a day, inflow versus outflow.

Christophe, Numa, and I worked out a rough rotation: two of us on duty for an eight hour shift, with one of us off. If we were extra-busy, which we usually were, everybody kept going. If things slowed down, one could rest by the fire. During the day, and for much of the night, the tents were uninhabitable because of the suffocating heat; the doors and windows laced tightly shut to keep out the armies of flies. We had to make constant rounds to check on IVs, hang up new bags, see that there was enough dry sand under the patient to soak up the outflow, and help drag away the dead to make new places for the living. At night we worked by flashlight and a few spirit lanterns, which we hung from the cross-poles. They reminded me of the four humors which formed all of Aristotle's universe: fire, air, water, earth. Our setting, and our actions, were about as basic as that.

And the flies. Where could they come from in such numbers? They were everywhere. Crawling in the excrement, buzzing at the mouths and eyes of the patients. Hiding in the thatch. Swooping into the food bowls of the relatives. They crawled up your wrist as you tried to insert an intravenous line or cut down on a collapsed vein, flew about your face as you walked from one patient to another. The flies often helped you distinguish the moribund but alive patient from the newly dead: when you saw them walking, undisturbed, over the whites of an opened eye, you knew the patient was gone.

At night, the flies were less visible and less active, but they were there. The banquet was still spread before them. If you had been careless, and they had found a way into your tent during daylight, they would emerge as you tried to get a few hours sleep, crawling on your skin or sleeping bag, reaching for your face.

Since Chad I have never again been comfortable with flies, even when they are in numbers small enough to kill. If you sit with me on my summer patio, over a glass of wine or a sandwich lunch, and if you are a careful observer, you will see me move slightly back from the table as a single fly explores the vicinity of the food. I don't like the sound of them, nor a smell that my faulty memory attributes to them, an odor that they themselves do not possess.

There was only one time of day when we could escape the flies. In the half-hour just before and after dawn, there was a hint of coolness in the air, a faint pink in the east that was soon to become a furnace of orange. There were very few large trees in the vicinity of the field hospital, but there was one giant baobab hung with weaver birds' nests off by itself. I would try to stand under it for a few moments just before dawn each morning, catching a hint of breeze, a wisp of coolness, and the temporary absence of the flies. Then the sun would rise, warming the air, and the flies would be there again.

Sometimes the Young Chinese Soldier would stand there with me in the pre-dawn half-light. He would never say a word, nor look at me directly, just stand there next to me, smoking a cigarette, and then turn and wander off into the bush.

The patients were mostly anonymous to us, too sick to have any interaction with, mumbling in a language that I did not understand. They came, they went, especially as the pressure of numbers rose. But among them there was one woman whose face I will not forget.

She was of indeterminate age and looked to be in the second trimester of pregnancy. She was as sick as most, but no sicker than many. For reasons that we never discussed, and probably could not have expressed, Christophe, Numa, and I wordlessly decided that we were determined to pull her through. When you came on shift, likely as not the first thing you would ask about was, "How is the pregnant woman doing?"

When you went off shift, she would usually be the last patient you looked after. In some way, I think she was our barometer as to whether sanity could be restored to our little world, whether life could indeed come again out of all this death.

For a day or so, we thought we were keeping up the pace with her. In terms of rehydration, and the slowing of diarrhea, she looked to be keeping ahead of the curve. And then, without warning, she aborted. So weak that she did not struggle or even cry out, we found the bloody mess between her legs in the sand. The next morning, when I came on shift and went first to her, there was another patient lying in her place. I asked Numa what had happened, though I knew full well. For once, he said nothing, just looked at me. We continued on our rounds.

Christophe and Numa had insisted that I take a separate sleeping tent but we messed together, usually in their larger tent. Meals were mostly a doughy ball made from millet flour with whatever sauce could be scraped together and additions from the dry rations I had brought with me. We drank water from the IV fluid bags. I had, among my rations, several cans of fruit in syrup. One night, unable to restrain myself, I gulped an entire can of peaches down by myself, in secret, alone in my tent. I felt great shame, and disgust at my personal weakness. I think that Christophe and Numa knew, but they never mentioned it.

At night, off to the northwest of our hospital, we could see the orange flickering of groups of large lines of fires, stark against the black skies, and setting the bright stars a-shimmering with their heat. Numa explained to me, "The villagers believe that they must burn their houses and their fields to rid themselves of the evil of this plague."

"But," I asked, "what will they do for food this winter if there are no crops?"

Christophe just looked at me, and shrugged. Then he turned, and gestured at the patients silent beneath the thatch, the murmuring groups of relatives huddled by their cookfires.

Burning fields and villages by night, truckloads of the soon-to-be-dead and the recently dead by day. I knew that, awake or asleep, I was in the landscape of hell, a canvas painted by Heironymus Bosch.

One evening a mobile vaccination team stopped by to visit Christophe and Numa. The team of four consisted of themselves and a dusty, rickety truck, their personal gear and supplies, and a small kerosene-fired refrigerator full of vaccine. As the four of them wearily swung down from the cab and the truck-bed, it was evident that they were old friends of the two field hospital nurses. Their burdens seemed to lighten as they embraced each other, gossiping and laughing with the mutual feigned insults that are the staple of comrades in the field. With me, they were initially more reserved, formal, even wary. Then Christophe muttered something, there was a great burst of laughter, and they surrounded me, relaxed, chattering words I could not comprehend but understood as a ribald acceptance.

They had brought along what remained of a small bush-gazelle, and cooked it up with our *boule* and spicy sauce as if it were a king's banquet. Unable to understand much of their multi-lingual banter, I sat back from the fire until my eyes closed, then excused myself and went to my tent. They talked and smoked late into the night. I could see them silhouetted against the rising sparks of the fire when I got up to check on the patients and I could hear Christophe and Numa move under the thatch shelter as they made rounds several times during the night. When I awoke before dawn, the visitors were gone. Numa said, "They say that things are very bad in the villages near here and that there is never enough vaccine. Many people do not live long enough for the trucks to bring them here. Many others leave the villages and wander off into the bush. But they also say that the epidemic seems to be slowing and that they have hope that it will not move much further east into the country, or south towards Fort Lamy. Perhaps, *mon Docteur*, we shall have luck after all. Hope and luck, that is what we need, is it not so?"

"That, and the strength to keep going, my friend," I answered. "Let's go make rounds." We each grabbed some bags of fluid and went to discover who was still alive.

The trucks that visited us twice or more a day to deliver to us their human cargo, living and dead, and to take from us only the dead were manned by young French soldiers, both conscripts and professionals. They had been assigned to the "cholera duty" from their regular postings in the desert north, where a nasty and unheralded war was going on between the government of Chad, and rebels supported by Libya. Aiding one side, Libyan irregulars. Aiding the other, French Army and Legionnaires.

When they learned that I was an American who spoke some French, they first asked me to ride with them one morning on their rounds. Thinking that I might be of some help, I threw my medical bag onto a truck and climbed in. One of the French soldiers, a medical corpsman, took my place to assist Christophe and Numa.

I encountered a landscape of such desolation as to beggar description. The land was parched, the sky cloudless, the sun searing, the fields untended if not burned black. The villages, reached by dirt track or direct through the bush, were mostly empty, their inhabitants having fled into the bush (to where?), except for those already ill and too weak to flee. In a few villages, the dead lay unburied, and in those villages, the dogs were no longer emaciated.

When we passed through those few villages as yet unaffected by the cholera, the usual extreme poverty of the inhabitants looked to us like great wealth compared with those villages that were burned-out husks. And, as we circled further and further east, loading up the trucks with the sick as we went, we saw the decreasing gradient of the epidemic's impact. As for my medical bag, I might just as well have left it back at the field hospital. There was not time to stop, nor really anything useful for me to do, except to help the soldiers load the sick into one truck and the dead into the other.

In the middle of my second week, as the flood of patients was beginning to slow down, the young French lieutenant who was in command of the truck detail asked if I would come to their camp and take lunch with them. His invitation to *prenez le déjeuner 'vec nous* was phrased as if we were to meet at some Parisian bistro. I accepted and was given directions, and noon as the arrival time.

The French camp was about fifteen kilometers from us with only a few dirt-track turns, a short stretch of bush-whacking, and a dry gulley showing on the hand-drawn map he left with me. I packed up a few cans of my remaining rations as a gift, made sure I had drinking water, flashlights, a spare can of petrol, and sand-tracks and shovel in my truck, and set off.

I arrived uneventfully, was welcomed and shown around the tent cluster and motor pool, and we squatted down in one of the larger tents for our meal.

Ah, the French. The food, a combination of military rations and supplements from some far-off town, was a welcome relief from my Chadian *boule*. And there was cheese (if dry), and bread (if hard), and even red wine (if coarse). We talked of France, of America, and of Chad. Like most young soldiers, they despised the country they were in, and wanted only to go home. When I asked them which was worse, rear-echelon work in the north, or cholera duty here, they looked at each other, and then one young soldier, who looked to be about eighteen, spat in the sand and said, *"Aucune différence"* (pretty much the same). *"Ou nous brûlons les villages, ou les gars, ils brûlent les villages eux-memes"* (either we burn down the villages, or those guys burn down the villages themselves).

I thanked them for their hospitality and headed back to my hospital.

From the trip coming out, I thought that I could save a little time by cutting in advance into the sandy gully, maybe take two or three kilometers off the journey, and I was in a hurry to get back. I cracked through some dry brush, got down onto the gully floor, and then realized I had made a mistake as the surface turned into a patch of looser and looser sand, and the gully walls rose to a height of eight or ten feet. I must have wandered into the sandy dry remnant of an ancient pool.

The wheels of the truck began to spin and the narrow passage allowed no significant room for maneuver. I tried to go a little faster, cutting my front wheels right and left, but soon I was trapped. I resisted the panicky urge to gun the engine, knowing it would drive my wheels, front and back, deeper into the sand, and stopped to have a look around.

I was caught in dry sand nearly up to the axles, front and rear. Any attempt to dig out would be futile. I tried sliding the sand-tracks (lengths of metal airfield matting that provide a hard surface) under the rear wheels, but that only drove the front wheels deeper, and I was reluctant to accelerate that process.

There was one spindly, but solid-enough looking tree on the edge of the gully above me to the left, and about thirty feet away. I drew out the chain and hook from the winch on the front bumper of the truck. It fell short by about four or five feet.

Well, I wasn't going to get myself out of there. If I had my hundred feet of parachute cord, I might double it over three or four times and make a loop around that tree that would be long enough and strong enough for me to reach with the hook from the winch's chain. But I didn't have the parachute cord. Maybe I could cut off the top of the tree, taking off the truck motor's fan belt, and looping it over the tree trunk to connect with the chain but, no, that wouldn't be long enough. Besides, if I broke the fan belt in the process, I would only be in bigger trouble. I'd searched three or four times in the truck and couldn't find extra rope or chain.

The obvious answer was to walk out to either the field hospital or the French camp for help and an extension to the winch chain. The French camp was closer and I could be sure to get there by following my fresh tire tracks. But they were likely to be out on their own rounds, though I could surely appropriate a rope from somewhere in the camp and explain later. So, back to the French camp it would have to be, a long, dusty, hot, and thirsty walk. I would have plenty of time before dark, I doubted there were any dangerous large animals about, and I could watch carefully for snakes.

He appeared at the edge of the gully, in the way that Africans have of appearing suddenly in the bush. Not there, and then there, silently.

He was as skinny as the long straight stick he carried in one hand. In the other he held an old lidless tin can, which probably had originally contained a quart of motor oil. His age was somewhere between twenty and fifty; I couldn't tell. Straight narrow nose, dark rheumy eyes, thin lips. His skin was dark and lined and leathery, and his bare feet were scarred and callused. His only clothing was a pair of tattered and stained short pants, once khaki, which were held up by a cotton string around the waist, the string itself broken and re-tied together several times.

And, he was smiling. He said not a word, just nodded his head up and down several times, and then held up his hand, dropping the stick, fingers spread and palm out and pushing toward me in the unmistakable gesture for "Wait." Then, he disappeared.

I took him at his word, or rather at his gesture, and sat down inside the truck for shade, doors left open to catch the non-existent breeze.

Thirty minutes later, he appeared again. This time he had, hanging around his neck like the coils of a python, a length of rusty log chain. He descended the gully wall and held the tin can out to me. It was filled with murky water, flecks of rust from the can drifting on its surface. I would not reject his hospitality, so I took a small sip, lips tight together, and then handed it back to him for his turn to drink. He drained the can, licked his lips, and motioned to me to follow him.

We slung the length of chain around the tree, down close to the ground for greater strength. Then we threaded the winch hook through the links of both ends, with several feet to spare, replaced the sand-tracks under the rear wheels, cranked up the motor and the winch, and pulled ourselves out of there in about thirty seconds, sand spewing behind the truck, out of the loose patch and onto firmer surface.

We retrieved the sand-tracks and the log chain, and took in the winch chain on the drum. My rescuer jumped into the front seat beside me, motioning me onward with a flicking of his wrist and open hand, palm down, until the gully walls fell away and we could exit onto the firm surface of the bush. Then he put his hand up for me to stop. He laid his hand upon my shoulder, then opened the door and stepped out. I signed to him that he could travel on with me; he shook his head. I offered him money; he pushed it gently away.

This man, with a stick, and a rusty tin can, and a length of chain, smiled again, and walked silently off into the bush in the direction from which he had come.

In Africa, the obligation to give assistance to a traveler is an ancient and a sacred one.

By the middle of the second week, we had sensed that the flow of patients was beginning to slow. We weren't keeping any sort of records or tally as we went about our monotonous and exhausting tasks, but there was a definite change of pace. The numbers of sand-spaces occupied under the thatch stopped climbing at somewhere over a hundred, then began to decline: ninety, eighty, back up to more than ninety, and then a slow downwards creep. Even more importantly, as happens with most epidemics, the new patients now seemed less acutely- and desperately-ill than earlier ones had been.

Passing vaccination teams confirmed for us that the tide was ebbing and the French Army trucks brought smaller loads, both living and dead, as well as bearing less dead away from us. It was clear by the middle of the second week that the epidemic had crested and was slowly waning. Probably more important in this process than the efforts of the vaccination teams were more "natural" forces: the sparseness of population and the increasing dryness of the landscape as one went east further into Chad, the flight of people to the east even before the epidemic reached them. Where had they gone? How many died in the bush, of hunger, thirst, or cholera itself? Perhaps, in a way, the tribal wisdom had been correct: burning the fields and villages, and thus forcing the people to scatter, may have broken the back of the epidemic. There were no towns of any size in the area. It looked as if, as was true in the event, Fort Lamy, a hundred kilometers to the south, would be spared.

And then, as our load of cholera patients began to decline, by the end of the second week, the children began to die.

Always balanced on that knife-edge of malnutrition, malaria, parasitic infestations, and other infections, those children in the surrounding villages whose mothers had died of cholera were now thrown off that knife-edge. For the nursing infants, especially, there were few healthy women who were not themselves malnourished, nursing infants of their own. The grandmothers' breasts were dry. And so more and more infants were brought to our station, I dare not call it a hospital in this context, with coughs and non-cholera diarrhea, with recurrences of malaria, with no specific conditions other than a profound and abrupt descent into acute starvation. The men and the old women held them out to us, but there was little we could do for them except to provide a small ration of millet gruel, which in many cases was not enough. The small supply of medicines from my medical bag was totally inadequate, and soon exhausted, to little benefit. There was nothing else. So we looked for wet-nurses, younger grandmothers, did our best, and watched them die. I thought often of what the coming winter would bring, with few crops left standing in the fields.

Late in the third week, Watel Bondo came through by Army helicopter. He looked exhausted. I suppose we all looked exhausted. The word was passed that we could abandon the field hospital and withdraw.

Before we burned it, I walked through the pole and thatch structure, the sand beneath my feet now dry, the central fire extinguished. The relatives' camp was empty, a metal pan or two left lying in the tall grass. A faint breeze rustled the thatch, and I could hear again the moans, and grunts, and whispers of the ghosts who had lain beneath it. Even the flies had mostly gone.

A truck came through to pick up the folded tents and the mountain of intravenous fluid, much smaller now than it had been. I was to take Christophe and Numa back to Fort Lamy. We piled the debris of our supplies under the thatched structure and set it ablaze. We stood together and watched until nothing but ash remained. Then Christophe and Numa jumped into the bed of my truck, I turned the ignition key, and we rolled south and west, into a land where the cholera had not come.

We said our goodbyes in front of the Ministry of Health. There really wasn't much to say; we had lived through the experience together, and now it was done. They would spend a few days in Fort Lamy and then be assigned to the mobile disease control teams, circling endlessly through the vast wastes of Chad, always short of petrol, vaccines, and medicines. But never, not my friends Christophe and Numa, never short of hope, nor of luck.

Watel Bondo was much too busy to say much more than a brief thank-you and a briefer goodbye. We agreed that we would see each other in a few months when things quieted down and I paid a return visit to Chad. But, in the end, it didn't work out that way.

I turned my truck and other gear back in at the Embassy. Jake took one look at me and dragged me off to his veranda, where I consumed four Cokes in a row, without waiting for ice. That was before the shower, and before the clean sheets. Next morning, I had more Coke for breakfast, and fresh papaya, with lemon, and fried eggs, and toast, and butter, and jam, and strong rich coffee. The dream began to fade. As I flew over the empty spaces of southern Chad and northern Cameroon, it faded further still. By the time I reached home in Yaoundé, it was all in the past.

Eight months later, back in the States, I saw a small item in the *New York Times*. Dr. Watel Bondo, my friend the "New Man of Africa," had fled to Paris, in open opposition to the government of Francois Tombalbaye. He gave a speech announcing the formation of a new political party.

Two men described as European had stepped out of the crowd and shot him to death, firing six times at close range, and disappearing back into the resulting confusion. No one was ever found, or charged.

EPILOGUE

"You cannot step twice into the same river,
for other waters and yet others, go ever flowing on."
—Heraclitus, c.540–c.480 B.C.

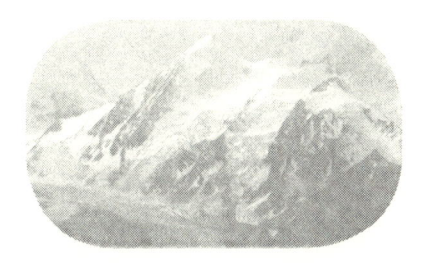

Though the river we have once traversed stays always unchanged in our memory, it never remains the same river in our dreams, nor from instant to instant in its own tangible existence.

Time has not been kind to the lands of the River of Stone and the River of Sand.

Nepal, whose theocratic monarchy once seemed to me in the 1960s to be relatively benign, if paternalistic, at the turn of the 21st Century was crushed between a despotic king, himself maintained by the army, and a demented Maoist rebellion reminiscent of Peru's Shining Path. Peasants were abused and murdered by both sides, the economic engine of tourism lay in shambles. A near-revolution that saw the Maoists gain by politics what they could not gain by terrorism brought down the king to powerlessness. The Maoists gathered into cantonments where their arms were under lock and key (but they retained the keys). A new constitution abolished the monarchy, and installed a floundering multi-party legislature in which the Maoists, who currently label themselves "capitalists, "seem to hold a whip hand. The surrounding giants, India and China, appear to feel that they have little at stake in the well-being of Nepal. They may learn otherwise should the fragile government collapse in the chaos of revolution, or should the Maoist insurgency recur and spill over into India's borderlands. As for the rest of the world, it seems to echo Dolma's remark, concerning the boy "of little significance."

Dolma and his countrymen still wait, and the other powers, those "of significance," find it most convenient to forget, or avert their eyes from, the continuing Chinese rape of Tibet. Pious statements and garlands of flowers shower upon the Dalai Lama from far and wide, but little real interest is exhibited in the fate of the people of Tibet. China continues its widespread destruction of the tangible and intangible treasures of Tibet, whose people spring from a different ethnicity, different religions, and a different culture. Mass planned, if not forced, in-migration of Han Chinese into Tibet abets the disappearance of what was once there. With the ascendancy of China on the world stage, there seems little hope for Dolma and his subjugated brothers and sisters.

As for Africa, both West and East: poor Africa. In the first decade following independence, a glowing, if modest, optimism regarding Africa's development was exemplified for me by Dr. Bondo, the "New Man of Africa." Whether Watel Bondo was assassinated by French or Chadian hirelings, by Europe or his own Africa, makes little difference. That former optimism has now mostly been extinguished in orgies of corruption, famine, plagues and other "natural" disasters, and in warfare, brutality, and genocide on a scale that, I believe, was never known in earlier times in "Darkest" Africa. The Great Powers strut, the United Nations postures, politicians on the Continent fill their filthy hands at the trough, and Africa sinks ever deeper into poverty.

Should you think that these are the fantasies and grumblings of a young man grown old, I say to you, "Go and look for yourselves."

The Science of Medicine that I struggled to learn as a young doctor in Africa and Asia three and four decades ago, is far eclipsed by the science of medicine as it is today. The revolution of molecular biology and the information power of the computer have given the young and not-so-young doctors of today knowledge and capabilities that were beyond our wildest imaginings in 1963, when I graduated from medical school and began my internship. It is even arguable that medicine has changed more in the past half-century than it changed in the half-century before that. What is certain is that the pace of change is steadily increasing, and that the next half-century will produce even greater wonders.

And yet, with every great advance and discovery, a next onion-layer of mystery and challenge is revealed, each solution leading to the uncovering of a new problem, what Rene Dubos called "The Mirage of Health." There have also been many significant setbacks: the challenge of organisms resistant to all current therapy, the emergence of new and fearsome global diseases, the resurgence of mass infectious disease, the specter of willful use of bioweapons, the rise of "diseases of affluence," and the many, and largely unknown, health effects of the desecration of our planetary environment.

So I think it is somewhat of an open question as to whether we, physicians and citizens, are further ahead or behind in the ongoing struggle for human health, whether in Kathmandu, Chad, or New York.

And what of the Art of Medicine? Here, I think, on balance it remains as it has been since the time of Hippocrates, and doubtless even before. The forms and contexts change, the scandals and outrages of the day come and go. But I believe that the innate seed of caring that urges young people to become physicians and nurses is as it always was, and stays with most of those individuals even as they are tempered, rewarded, and battered by life and society's vicissitudes. If there is one thing that keeps me optimistic, it is that belief.

As for me, there have been many rivers to cross since those of Stone and of Sand. Some have flowed full and bountiful, between banks of green meadows. A few have been bitter trickles, wandering across alkali flats in lands of no rain. And some have been turbulent, tempestuous, throwing spray and spume as high as the moon. These latter have been the ones I've loved best.

I do believe that "you cannot step twice into the same river," and that, "once crossed, there are borders you cannot go back across again." But the greater mystery for me is: "Who is the you whose life traverses those passages?" Is it forever the same "you," whose innate and predetermined nature is merely unfolded by experience? Or is it a more malleable, unprogrammed "you," who, immersed in the river of life, changes, adds, and subtracts its character and qualities because of that flow?

Perhaps it does not matter much, but I would surely like to know.

The Young Chinese Soldier still comes to me in dreams, silent as always, but he comes less often now. It is Pemba whom I see more often these nights, not because of what my colleagues and I did up on the Tibetan frontier, but because of what Pemba symbolizes: the importance of putting aside false distinctions of "significance."

I would dearly love to see those Khamba bandits again, and Madame Delphine, and most of all Christophe and Numa, but I know I never will. They are the heroes of this world, they and the barefoot porters, and the match-stick mechanic, and the skinny man with the log chain. They are souls of full measure, ready to give much, and expecting little in return. It is they who understand "significance."

And, of course, the rivers and the mountains still abide, and are there for us to cross and to climb. What would the world be, how would life go on, what would we do, without them?